LIVING *from the* INSIDE OUT

LIVING *from the* INSIDE OUT

HOW TO BECOME A MODERN-DAY WONDER WOMAN

Alison Wheeler

First published in 2022 by Dean Publishing
PO Box 119
Mt. Macedon, Victoria, 3441
Australia
deanpublishing.com

DEAN PUBLISHING

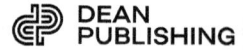

Cataloguing-in-Publication Data
National Library of Australia
Title: Living From The Inside Out — How To Become A Modern-Day Wonder Woman
Edition: 1st edn
ISBN: 978-1-925452-46-4
Category: Self-help/Personal Growth/Memoir

Dedication

To my husband, who is steadfast in his belief and insight.
You are the person I can trust and bounce all my crazy
thoughts off.

To my daughter—I hope I live as an inspiration
to you each and every day.

To my dad—you are no longer here with us, but
you were foundational in me becoming all I am today
and the reason I have a ferocious attitude towards
achieving the next level.

To my mum—you demonstrate what love is and
what it means to be a mum, and for that—
I am so thankful.

Alison is sharing more in her INTERACTIVE book.

See exclusive downloads, videos, audios and photos.

DOWNLOAD it for free at deanpublishing.com/alisonwheeler

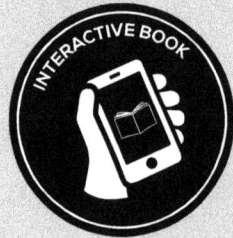

INTERACTIVE BOOK

CONTENTS

How to best use this book

Welcome to my book fellow modern-day wonder women,

No doubt you have a super busy life and you're possibly wondering how can you get the most value out of this book and use your time wisely. Here are my top tips:

- Read a chapter and then pause
- Complete the exercises for that specific chapter
(grab yourself the workbook – so you can write all over it)
- Take action as outlined in the book
- Watch the interactive videos for that chapter

Once you have implemented the above, then move onto the next chapter. You aren't required to hurry, just move through the book at a pace that feels right to you, chapter by chapter. It's best to use this book as a companion and you may wish to go over some exercises more than once.

Most of all, enjoy the journey.

Purpose of this book

I have always been driven, maybe by a level of dissatisfaction, but I assume it's mainly from an innate curiosity for what is possible. This curiosity has meant that I have achieved a lot in my life, but still couldn't satisfy something inside. That led to burnout and all sorts of issues. But most of all, it led to feeling unworthy. I'm so grateful that with the right knowledge and insight, I got to look at this unworthiness and overcome it.

My wish for you beautiful reader, is that this book can assist you to find and accept your worthiness, and believe deeply in yourself and your own unique superpowers. You are more gifted and able than you may ever believe.

I believe in you.

Alison

Listen to a special Welcome video by Alison in the bonus interactive book. Go to **deanpublishing.com/alisonwheeler**

INTRODUCTION

Full Circle

LOSING MYSELF TO FIND MYSELF

Looking back over my life to where I am now, I realise the journey I've been on was leading me to this very point. A stage in my life where I finally feel comfortable with who I am and where I am. I am proud to call myself a successful businesswoman, wife and mother, and I'm doing something I absolutely love—helping people realise their true potential.

Seeing my clients learn, grow and make positive changes to their lives and fulfil their dreams is incredibly satisfying and I love it!

Reaching this point has not been all smooth sailing and I have taken many different paths along the way. However, the challenges I've had to overcome and the lessons I've learnt in doing so have made me who I am today and I'm grateful for every single one. The challenges have filled me with new inner resources and have provided me with a resilient skillset. I'm now blessed to be able to share my skillset to pay it forward and help others.

Throughout this book, I would like to share my personal journey with you and be open about the lessons I gathered along the journey. As Steve Jobs once said, "You can't connect the dots looking forward; you can only connect them looking backwards." I agree. It's only in reflecting back that I can now see that a bigger destiny was unfolding and every thing that happened (or didn't happen) was for a reason. And that reason was me. So I could become the person I was destined to be; to reach my full potential. And you can't do that with only successes, it takes trials and challenges to reach your best.

Essentially, this is why I wrote this book. So you, the reader, could take charge of your life and express your true self in all its exquisite glory. So you could reach the heights of your own potential and discover new strengths within yourself.

You see, I believe who you are—your true self—isn't fixed at birth. We take different roads in life in order to develop, grow and discover all aspects of ourselves. Life is about becoming who we are, creating ourselves from the inside-out, and developing our potential along the way. As Deepak Chopra said,: "The most creative act you will ever undertake is the act of creating yourself."

And although it took me many years and a great deal of soul searching, to peel back the layers and realise that being my true self was perfectly okay, the journey was certainly worth it. And I can guarantee it will be worth it for you too. This is why I wrote this book.

You see, no matter how windy and crazy the road may seem at times, if you remain focused on what you want and keep congruent with your values and dreams—then, you will awaken your true potential and reach heights that will astound you.

When you are inspired by some great purpose, some extraordinary project, all your thoughts break their bonds; Your mind transcends limitations, your consciousness expands in every direction, and you find yourself in a new, great and wonderful world. Dormant forces, faculties and talents become alive, and you discover yourself to be a greater person by far than you ever dreamed yourself to be.[1]

THE EARLY YEARS

I was born in Takapuna New Zealand, on the 23rd of May 1979, the youngest of three girls. My father's side was Portuguese, and my mother's was Scottish.

Whilst my sisters inherited the blue eyes and blonde hair from my mother's side, I was the little girl with dark hair and green eyes, from my father's side.

My parents were wonderful, hardworking people who did everything they possibly could to give my sisters and I the best possible start in life. We were a very close family and I have happy childhood memories.

While we were growing up, my parents ran holiday parks and for my sisters and me, this was a wonderfully carefree time. We had ample freedom and spent a lot of our time outside exploring and playing with the other children who were holidaying there.

However, from time to time our family's happy life was disrupted by my father's serious health issues. When I was around three or four years old, my father had to be on dialysis because his kidneys had failed. Although he was able to do this treatment at home, it meant there would be periods where our lives revolved around his treatment. As a young child, to see my strong, hardworking father, incapacitated during these times was difficult for me to understand. It certainly impacted my sisters and I.

During those early years we were living with my grandparents so fortunately my mother had extra support. They were such an important and much-loved part of my life, especially my grandmother.

After Dad had his first successful kidney transplant his health improved and life returned to some normality.

When I was around six years old, my grandparents decided to sell the holiday park my parents were working in, so we moved to the town of Cambridge, where my parents managed another holiday park.

Several years later, my father's kidney transplant failed and he had to undergo another one, which involved a lengthy hospital stay.

I remember how shocking it was to come home and find out my father wasn't there because he'd been taken away by ambulance and that we'd have to go through all the trauma again. Our grandparents were also no longer living with us, so my mother no longer had that extra support.

Thankfully, after my father's second kidney transplant, he was well again and able to return to his much-loved sport of running. Dad was very good at running and went on to represent New Zealand in the Transplant Games. Dad's athletic ability and love of competition certainly rubbed off on me.

Although, back then, I didn't really know what I wanted to be when I grew up, I was incredibly self-driven and determined to achieve the very best at whatever I chose. I naturally had very high expectations of myself and was never one to settle for second best. To be honest, I'm not sure where this intense energy came from, nor did my parents. Perhaps, deep down, I knew I was destined for something pretty amazing.

Growing up, I thought that everyone else had the same attitude to life as I did, but I was wrong., I learnt early on that I really didn't fit the mould of how a young girl was expected to be. Back in those days boys and girls were seen in very traditional and stereotypical ways and I didn't fit that stereotype. Girls were supposed to be quiet, sweet and play certain games. Boys were considered more outdoorsy and sporty than girls. Although these archaic ideas aren't true, they were certainly projected in society at the time.

I wasn't the 'typical girl'. I was incredibly driven, with endless amounts of energy, always striving to excel, particularly in sport and school, and my fierce determination made people uncomfortable, and made it difficult for me to find my place in the world.

I was lucky that both my parents were athletic and had already introduced me to sports. A place I felt comfortable in. I loved everything about it. I loved the competition, the effort, the trying, the failing and the winning. It was my peaceful place and it gave me a sense of belonging.

I started in athletics around age seven, following the same path as my father, and later went on to netball and rowing. You name it and I signed myself up for it. Whilst my parents were very encouraging and supportive, they never pushed me. In fact, I was the one pushing myself. They used to say to me—"You need to calm down and slow down. Why are you driving yourself so much? You'll drive yourself into an early grave!"

But this was just who I was, and I approached everything in my life with the same drive and determination. Striving to be the best, I pushed my young body hard and injured my Achilles tendon at the age of nine. Not being able to compete was incredibly hard for me. I hated being a spectator! Thanks to a lot of physio and, years later, a reconstruction, the injury did heal. In retrospect, that taught me, with determination, it's always possible to find a solution.

All these sporting activities did however cost money, and although my parents worked very hard, often seven days a week, there was little left over for extras. I realised from a young age if I wanted extra things, I had to figure out how to do that on my own.

From around the age of ten or eleven I was doing whatever jobs I could, including a paper round and a cleaning job. I also worked in a service station at the local supermarket, and made crafts with my grandmother to sell. I did whatever I could to raise the money I needed, whether it was for a new bike, or to pay for my sport. I didn't realise it at the time but I was starting to build an attitude of "If it's meant to be, it's up to me." A mindset of getting things for myself and developing the persistence to achieve my goals.

"THE OPPORTUNITY OF A LIFETIME IS TO PICK YOURSELF.
QUIT WAITING TO GET PICKED; QUIT WAITING
FOR SOMEONE TO GIVE YOU PERMISSION; QUIT
WAITING FOR SOMEONE TO SAY YOU ARE
OFFICIALLY QUALIFIED...AND PICK YOURSELF."
SETH GODIN

MY TEEN YEARS

As I shared, as a child, I figured the world was a pretty straightforward place and that everyone thought like I did. It was only when I started secondary school that I began to realise people didn't think the same way as me, in fact they thought very differently. It became obvious that if I wasn't prepared to conform to the norm, then life was going to be uncomfortable.

Although I loved certain aspects of school and was a good student, socially I found it very challenging and discovered how nasty kids could be. The kids at school really couldn't figure me out because I didn't fit into a specific clique, which is what was important at the school I attended and a signature of teenage peer groups.

My peers criticised me for being too driven—as if there was something wrong with that. I ended up carrying those criticisms and those labels throughout my young adult life, desperately trying to work out where I actually fitted in.

I found an outlet, an escape of sorts, in rowing. I poured myself into rowing because it was an activity and outlet where I felt safe but this involved a huge amount of commitment and an intense training regime, both before and after school.

I pushed myself hard and achieved a lot of success. I competed at a National level and logged up a number of impressive awards. I was later selected to trial for the Under 19s New Zealand team and also awarded the school's Cambridge High School Laurel Award.

I enjoyed pushing my limits and achieving, however it came at a price. My dedication resulted in me often pushing my limits to a breaking point.

Between the bullying issues at school and my 'go hard' attitude to sport, I ended up contracting glandular fever in my second last year at school.

The stress from the bullying I was being subjected to at school, combined with the added pressure of the training I was doing, eventually led to my body giving me a very strong message that my reserves were running low. I was diagnosed with glandular fever and was away from school for three months.

When I recovered and was well enough to eventually return to school, I was shown little sympathy and my teachers just expected me to catch up with the work I'd missed over those three months. This only added to my stress.

HELL AND HEALING

Like many kids, before I went through puberty, I was tall and lean but then hormones kicked in and my body changed. Although I was still training at a high level, my body was changing and I was becoming bulkier. The change in my body felt strange and I guess for the first time in my life, I felt fat. The fact that other kids were noticing my weight and commenting on it, made me incredibly self-conscious.

This is the period in my life when my inner critic really started to take control. I had no idea how to fit in with the rest of the kids at school and now my body was changing, leading me to have a very distorted image of myself. I was battling on the inside. And although I wasn't totally aware of what all these emotions and body-shaming moments were triggering within me, looking back I can see this is where my battle with a serious eating disorder actually began.

After I graduated from secondary school, I went to Waikato University and then onto the University of Otago. I was studying Dietetics but also decided to apply to do army officer training during my university holidays. I was eighteen and looking forward to becoming independent.

I was always searching for the next challenge and the officer training certainly offered me that. There was also the added incentive of the army covering my university fees.

I would travel to Waiouru Army Camp to do my army officer training. It was demanding and rigorous, but it provided the challenge I craved.

At first, I found the training exhilarating and enjoyed the camaraderie between my fellow recruits. I pushed myself as hard as I possibly could, striving to be better and stronger than everyone else.

However, I soon worked out that attempting to stand out in the army was strongly discouraged and that it was all about group thinking. It was obvious that individuality and self-expression wasn't going to be developed in an environment where I was once again under pressure to conform and not buck the system.

During this time, my eating disorder was in full swing and was trying to keep up with my university studies. I wasn't coping with the pressure to manage everything and I began to question my choices—my choice of career and my decision to sign up for army officer training. I didn't want to continue with Dietetics at university because the course was not about people, it was about grinding things up. And on top of that, I was questioning the army officer training but knew I was contracted to complete it. I was literally spinning out of control because I didn't know who I was any more.

I was feeling increasingly desperate because I simply didn't know where I fitted in, or, for that matter, how to fit in. I was using food as a control mechanism for what felt like an out of control situation. I knew that the army environment wasn't going to provide me with what I really needed to flourish and I realised I had to withdraw from the army. This wasn't going to be easy as I had signed an agreement for several years.

During this period, my mental and physical health were beginning to spiral out of control, and I just couldn't cope with the real world anymore. My bulimia had become so serious that I really thought I was going to die. I rang Mum and begged her to come to Otago and bring me home, which she thankfully did.

So began a long period of healing my broken body and finding a way out of the terrible confusion and despair I was feeling. My eating disorder had taken me to the lowest and darkest point in my life and I needed to find my way out.

Fortunately, I was with my parents and had their love and support to help me through the dark days.

Throughout this period (which lasted several years) I had countless sessions with psychologists and psychiatrists and did a lot of self-reflection and introspection.

Throughout my healing journey, it occurred to me that my unhealthy obsession with controlling my eating was connected to my sense of powerlessness in other aspects of my life, in particular my confusion about trying to find my place in the world. As famous actor Susan Sarandon said publicly, "I think sometimes what happens is that all of this feeling out of control manifests itself in trying to control your body; whether it's an eating disorder or talking about getting your nose fixed, as if that's going to be the solution to all the pressure."

I eventually came to the conclusion that I was the only person who could fix me, and I needed to work out how to do this. I knew that I needed to find a permanent way to get out of this dangerous and destructive cycle of self-punishment. I needed to discover new parts of myself and nurture myself back to health.

Although each person's healing journey is different, for me, I had to want to get better first. I needed that internal drive within to fire on all cylinders. I need intrinsic motivation.

So I began to really work on myself and gradually started to feel a little less lost. I was beginning to reclaim a new part of myself; a part that no-one else could reach. A deeper part of myself was beginning to emerge.

MY TURNING POINT

The first step towards my recovery was making a fresh start by changing my university course from Dietetics to a Diploma in Fitness.

During my diploma I worked in the head injury unit of a rehabilitation hospital and through that I discovered Occupational Therapy. I found this to be an occupation that really intrigued me, so at the age of twenty, I transferred over to this.

Finding something I really enjoyed doing, helped me begin to put an end to the dreadful cycle of my eating disorder. However, I knew this was a complex and secretive disease that could claim me again, so I had to continue to be vigilant.

In 2004, after finishing my degree and gaining greater clarity about my direction, I moved to Australia and obtained further qualifications in soft tissue injury management from James Cook University, Townsville.

As part of my soft tissue training, I ended up volunteering in an Olympic weightlifting gym and that's where the next chapter of my life began. I was doing athlete assessments and helping the Olympic weightlifting team with their performance, and I met Paul—a weightlifting coach who had the same passion for sport as me.

We were both training and working with athletes, and we ended up spending a lot of time together. My personal interest in Olympic weightlifting was sparked and, with Paul's encouragement, I decided to pursue it. Naturally, I pursued it with vigour and determination and with Paul's support and advice, I ended up competing in Olympic weightlifting at a national level.

Paul was married when I first met him, although he and his wife were separated; so the beginning, our relationship was platonic. But as we got to know each other, we both realised there was a strong mutual attraction and deep connection. Paul decided he had to formally end his marriage before we could go any further in our relationship.

Paul and I had a special undeniable connection and we were prepared to go through whatever life threw at us together.

This was a tough time for both of us. Paul had the stress of managing a difficult divorce and, back in New Zealand, my father was diagnosed with stage four adrenal cancer. Being a kidney transplant recipient, my father was unable to have the standard cancer treatment and the doctors gave him three months to live.

My father proved the doctors wrong and survived another eighteen months, and, together with my mother, he was able to travel to Australia to see me. In fact, my parents even worked in Australia for a short time, managing a backpacker hostel, before returning home to New Zealand.

It was a time of dreadful anticipation because I knew my father wasn't going to recover and that any day, I may need to fly back home to be with him.

My amazingly strong dad who was such an important influence in my life, much throughout his life, finally passed away in 2004 at the age of 54. I was just so grateful Paul had the opportunity to meet him.

Looking back, it was amazing that Paul and I built such a great relationship through these tough times, but we did and the personal challenges we were both facing brought us closer together. We figured if we could get through this, we could survive anything.

As Paul was struggling with his divorce, a friend suggested he sign up to do a personal development course and I decided to sign up with him.

This was 2008 and this decision to do the course sparked another interest in me. Because it fell under the broader discipline of occupational therapy, both Paul and I started exploring the fascinating field of personal development, going on to enrol in various courses, including life coaching and neurolinguistic programming. I discovered that I loved everything about it and wanted to learn more.

I was still training at a high level with my weightlifting and decided I wanted to train for the Commonwealth Games, so life was pretty exciting.

Paul and I were now officially a couple and very committed to each other. He was keen to start a family, but I was focused on my training and achieving my goal of competing at the Commonwealth Games.

Paul accepted my decision and we thought that was that. However, something triggered my maternal instinct and I decided I really wanted to have a baby.

When I think back on this time, it was actually quite bizarre and hard to explain. I just knew I wanted to be pregnant, but it had to fit in with my training schedule. With the Games not far away, the window of opportunity was small. I told Paul that if we wanted to conceive, I would have to fall pregnant within the next three days. Amazingly, I did!

I enjoyed a healthy, easy pregnancy and was able to train throughout it. I did my last competition when I was six months pregnant and was training the morning I went into labour.

On the 19th of April 2009, our daughter Jasmine entered the world and a few months later Paul and I married in front of our families. We also did a naming ceremony for Jasmine the same day, so it was very special.

Motherhood was another major turning point in my life. I was now responsible for a tiny little human who was completely dependent on me. No one told me how difficult it would be transitioning to motherhood. I had always been so career-focused and was now running my own successful occupational therapy consultancy.

Motherhood was a complete change to my life which I felt quite unprepared for. It took me some time to find my feet as a mother, and it definitely triggered some questions about my identity and who I was. I now know that many mothers go through this transitory phase, but at the time I felt it was just me.

Around the same time Paul had started his own coaching and network marketing business, selling personal development products and events. He wanted me to get involved but at that stage I really wasn't interested. My focus was on being a mum.

I tried going back to my occupational therapy work but trying to juggle this with a new baby was proving difficult. I knew I had to find another way and I guess the answer was there right in front of me.

I could join the business with Paul and build it into a full-time career. This meant I would have the flexibility to be my own boss and be around for Jasmine and still help others. So Paul and I combined our efforts and poured our energy into parenting and business. I'm proud to say that we now have a highly successful business which allows us to enjoy a wonderful lifestyle.

We certainly work hard and are continuing to build our business, but we also have the freedom and flexibility to share as much quality time as we want with our growing daughter.

I am very proud of what we have achieved, and our business is going from strength to strength; recently achieving a record $213,000 USD a month in profit.

More importantly, I love using my time to pursue things that I'm passionate about. I have now been coaching people for over twelve years and

I love helping others change their lives.

As you can see from my journey, getting to where I am today has certainly had its challenges; it wasn't just a simple and straightforward journey.

In writing this book and sharing myself intimately, I have taken time to reflect on many of the important lessons I've learnt along the way. I'd love to share them with you in the hope they motivate and inspire you towards your dreams the same way they have propelled me forward. As the scholar Oliver Wendell Holmes once said, "Learn from the mistakes of others…You can't live long enough to make them all yourself!"

SUPERPOWER #1

Finding Your Okay Space Inside

"

COURAGE STARTS WITH SHOWING UP AND LETTING OURSELVES BE SEEN.

"

Brené Brown

Purpose

To understand that life is a journey
and we pick up and agree with a lot of
outside opinions and labels along the way.
Superpower 1 is about finding the courage
to peel these back and set your own
standards; to discover your self-worth and
values based on what is inside you, not
from what others have given you

You are braver than you think, and have
more value than you could ever imagine.

Check out Alison's personal video to
you, the reader, about Superpower 1
in the bonus interactive book. Go to
deanpublishing.com/alisonwheeler
to discover more.

"

WE CAN'T HELP
THE WAY
WE'RE BORN.
WE CAN'T HELP
WHAT WE ARE,
ONLY WHAT
WE CHOOSE
TO MAKE
FOR OURSELVES.

"

Wonder Woman: Warbringer

L ife teaches us many lessons along the way but perhaps this is the most important—the key to true inner strength and happiness is authenticity.

We can't help the way we're born, and the unique core traits that make us who we are, should be nurtured and celebrated.

As I have gone through life, I have found that being true to yourself often does not come easily. From a very young age, we learn that society expects us to conform to its expectations and that stepping outside the 'norm' comes with certain risks. The risk to be classified as different or weird, the risk to be criticised and ostracised. The risk to be labelled and judged. It's no wonder that stepping out the box of conformity makes people feel uneasy.

In order to fit in, we sometimes dull our potential and allow others to label us. We seek others' approval and validation instead of our own. We give away our power in order to conform. This leaves us feeling disempowered and unfulfilled because we are not being true to ourselves.

According to Buddhist teachings, if we have the courage to look at ourselves honestly, we are able to see both our flaws and basic goodness. This is known in the Buddhist tradition as our 'buddha-nature'. It involves letting go of our egos and getting in touch with our true selves.

Yet, how many of us have the courage to accept our true selves—both our strengths and imperfections? How many of us are truly unapologetic about who we are and comfortable in our own skins?

This is not just about feeling comfortable about our physical appearance, it's also about accepting those innate aspects of our personality and not feeling like we have to make apologies for being our authentic self. As Albert Einstein reminded us, "The person who follows the crowd will usually go no further than the crowd. The person who walks alone is likely to find himself in places no one has ever seen before."

Yet we aren't given this wisdom growing up. We often have to discover it ourselves. A common saying when I was growing up was, "Children should be seen and not heard."

Little girls, in particular, were expected to be compliant and quiet and differences were discouraged. As a result, I believe many young women, including myself, grew up thinking we were flawed in some way. I'm happy to see this change over time, but of course there's still a lot of room for improvement.

Society still inflicts massive amounts of silent social pressure on women. Women are often expected to do it all, and do it in a way that society deems 'acceptable'. The myriad of pressures range in the way we dress, look, behave, eat and even parent.

Although there are societal pressures on men too, I believe that they tend to have more leeway to make mistakes and are allowed to be more outwardly expressive, especially in the workplace.

In order to be ourselves and live authentically we must understand that the messages we received growing up and the societal pressures to conform shaped us in some way. However, as adults, we don't have to dance to their tune anymore, we can choose who and what influences us and pave our own path forward.

In other words, you don't have to participate in the past labels you were given by others. You can stop living the labels assigned by others and start living according to your true self. If you silently accept the labels others have assigned to you, then you're living inauthentically. I always encourage my clients to address any internal conflicts between living a life others expect them to live versus the life they want to live. If you have an internal conflict because you feel boxed by the expectations of others and can't be yourself, then you will need to address why you feel the need to gain others approval and validation. If every time you express yourself, and there's a fight within you because you are worried about what people will think about you, then there is some internal work that needs to be done.

When others label or criticise you, remember it's not necessarily about you. It often reveals more about them. Sometimes it can be because you're reflecting something they are missing within themselves.

Perhaps your kindness makes them uncomfortable because, deep down, they'd rather be a better person. Perhaps the fact you're so driven and goal orientated makes them feel uncomfortable because they've already given up on their own dreams.

The only way for insecure people to make themselves feel validated and comfortable within themselves, is to make what you're doing wrong—to invalidate it. That makes their world right and safe and means they don't have a reason to challenge it and change what needs to be changed.

There will always be critics and naysayers in this world. There will always be some people who find it their duty to assign blame and shame to others. Don't let these types of people define you. Don't let others decide who you are. Only you know who you really are; so be that person on purpose. Be yourself fully and don't make apologies for it. As perfectly said by Ralph Waldo Emerson, "To be yourself in a world that is constantly trying to make you something else is the greatest accomplishment."

PEELING OFF THE LAYERS

As I have shared, when I set out on my personal development journey, I genuinely thought there was something wrong with me. As a result, I allowed others to judge and label me, and tell me what was right for me. I allowed myself to be invalidated by other people's opinions on what I was supposed to do. Does this sound familiar?

As I began to understand how certain events and experiences had shaped me, I realised I wasn't actually broken—I didn't need fixing. There were just layers I needed to peel off, to reveal more of who I actually was. I needed to give myself permission to explore and express myself fully. To accept myself unconditionally.

In psychology the term, "Peeling back the layers" or "peeling back the onion" is simply a metaphor for unravelling the layers of yourself in the process of self-discovery. It's considered a gentle and slow way to peel back the hidden parts of yourself in order to allow your full self to emerge. This process can include reclaiming suppressed or underdeveloped parts of yourself, or discovering new parts that may have laid dormant or have never been awakened.

The reason this is so powerful is because it allows you to drop all the social masks and just relax into your true being. When you go through the process of peeling back the layers, you realise that what's left is simply you and that nobody else has that blueprint. You are a one-off! As Oprah

Winfrey said, "If you peel back the layers of your life—the frenzy, the noise—stillness is waiting. That stillness is you."

For me, that was a pretty exciting discovery. I also realised that peeling back the layers was going to be an ongoing process—requiring constant reflection and self-love. It wasn't a destination, it was a journey. So I didn't need to sprint at it, I just needed to stay with the unfolding process.

To be truly comfortable in my own skin, I needed to become my own best friend, regardless of how other people responded to me. That wasn't necessarily an easy road, but well worth the effort to travel it. It's also something I suggest often to my clients. I challenge them to be-friend themselves, to be there for themselves the same way they are there for other people.

Peeling back the layers means finding new places inside yourself bit by bit, layer by layer. Exploring your vulnerabilities and letting the light shine in.

In many ways, learning to love yourself for who you are and as you are is the most important healing journey you can take. It often leads to exciting discoveries too. Like this story I'd like to share.

When I was one-year-old, I suffered quite a serious burn. Our grandmother was looking after us and she was taking a roast chicken out of the oven and the bottom tray fell out. I was splashed by the very hot oil and ended up in hospital with third degree burns to my shoulder and back.

Once the burn healed it left quite a prominent scar and had to wear compression garments and had specialist appointments until I was eleven. Until the day she died my grandmother never forgave herself and was always urging me to put sunscreen on my scar.

When I met my husband, Paul, the scar was still very obvious. Now, this may sound seemingly impossible to many, but as I was going through my personal development journey, the more I explored my thinking and started 'cleaning up' my own mental environment, the entire colour and appearance of my scar began to change and gradually fade.

Even though there may be some plausible medical explanation for this change, I see it as a powerful, physical example of what happens when you do manage to find your okay space inside. When you get good with yourself, you heal yourself emotionally, but you can also heal physical aspects of yourself.

Louise Hay, the famous author of *You Can Heal Your Life* also discovered the same thing, when she healed her emotional wounds, she also healed her cancer-ridden body. She discovered the mind-body connection was a powerful and miraculous force. As Deepak Chopra said, "The mind and the body are like parallel universes. Anything that happens in the mental universe must leave tracks in the physical one."

My scar was my physical track, and the healing that was taking place on the inside was being seen on the outside.

Throughout the process of healing, I realised that I didn't need permission to be my true self, I actually needed to be more of my true self. But having this understanding and applying it to my everyday life were two different things. That, I'd have to learn.

I also discovered that success had to come from me, because you can't succeed like someone else. You have to create your own version of success—a success that reflects you and no one else.

These insights may sound cliché or obvious but let me assure you that living them is very different to understanding them. Living them is transformational.

DEVELOPING MY 'TEFLON' COATING

There's a common saying we fling around in society to try and 'help' people deal with criticism and rejection. It's recommended that we develop "a thicker skin".

Although, this can also be interpreted as "don't take things personally,"—it can also form layers of emotional detachment and 'blocking' our emotions. It can make us shut off from others and develop emotional walls to survive the brutal world we find ourselves in.

I was given this advice when I experienced some harsh bullying in high school. It was both personal and cruel and I felt quite alone. When I was growing up there was little, if any, understanding about the serious impact bullying can have on kids and my teachers offered little support. Bullying was seen as a part of growing up and accepted as 'what kids do'. You were simply expected to deal with it by developing a 'thicker skin' and becoming more resilient. So, I guess I did as I was told and developed a thicker skin. This was my way of coping and surviving my final few years of school.

I also found that, in retaliation to the bullying, to survive, I was becoming a bully myself. I remember thinking—*This is terrible. What am I doing? You can't take this out on other people. Why am I doing this?*

Looking back over this difficult period in my life, I don't really know why I was a target for the bullying. I guess it was because there were a lot of cliques and you were either in this group or that group. I remember, at the time, thinking—*This is dumb. I don't want to be in any of those groups, but where do I fit in?* I didn't think I was a nerd, but I guess, by definition I probably was. I also wasn't one of the popular kids because with my sport I didn't socialise much, so I didn't really fit in anywhere. I didn't have a label and that was a problem at my school. Labels were considered vital.

Looking back, although I did well at school, I don't think I achieved as much as I could have because of the bullying and constant pressure of trying to fit in.

To make things even worse, skin problems haunted me. During this time my skin broke out quite badly, which certainly didn't help with the bullying! I was prescribed a medication called Roaccutane, a popular acne treatment at the time.

One of the side effects is that it causes fragile skin. I was trialing for the New Zealand national rowing team at the time but had to pull out of the trials because I had literally ripped my hands to shreds from the oars. So much for 'developing a thicker skin!'

The 'build a thicker skin' advice was failing me. It wasn't until I returned back from my bout of glandular fever three months later and my teachers demanded that I catch up on the work that I had missed, that I figured some things aren't simply fixed by developing a tougher skin.

At this time, I remember begging my parents to send me to the local private school for the remainder of my last two years of school. Not only would it be a fresh start for me, it also happened to be an amazing rowing school, with state-of-the art facilities.

Unfortunately, there was no way my parents could afford the fees and I couldn't figure out a way to raise the funds myself. This meant I had to push myself through the final few years of high school whether I liked it or not. To say that I was grateful to finally graduate and move on is an understatement.

I find it sad that all these years later, bullying continues to be a serious issue in our schools. Kids are still being told to develop a thicker skin—an expression I have come to dislike because I think it sends out a message that to succeed in this world, you need to be hard and almost unfeeling.

While I agree we need to teach our children to be resilient, I prefer to use the term, 'Teflon coating'. Teflon coating is a term made famous in cookware due to its non-stick, non-reactive properties. With a Teflon coating, you're able to deflect negativity and criticism without letting it stick but you still retain the ability to connect and feel. This is a better alternative than rigidly blocking out, numbing or denying our feelings, as we all know that this can lead to a myriad of physical and psychological problems. With Teflon coating you still feel the temperature of your feelings and environment but you remain less reactive. You avoid blocking out the pain and stop pretending that it doesn't exist. Instead you work with the situation and stay connected to your feelings while developing the ability to not let sh*t stick.

TIPS TO DEVELOPING A TEFLON COATING

Developing a Teflon coating is a balancing act—you need to remain connected to your feelings without getting hooked by other people's emotional responses. You need to remain less reactive (like Teflon) to sudden triggers or changes.

For example, being criticised unfairly by someone could easily set the scene for being emotionally triggered. In the past, you may have dealt with this in one of two ways: either by getting upset and offended, or by developing a "thicker skin" and blocking the uncomfortable feelings. Developing a Teflon coating gives you a third option. Instead of getting upset or numbing out the feelings, you can simply label what is happening and stay less reactive. You can tell yourself, "They are criticising me unfairly and that reveals more about them than me." You can assess the situation without being hooked by it and erect healthy boundaries so you don't fall prey to their toxic behaviour. It's good to think of your Teflon coating as a healthy boundary, a coating that allows you to feel but also enables things to slip off and not stick.

> *"TO AVOID CRITICISM, SAY NOTHING,*
> *DO NOTHING, BE NOTHING."*
> ***ARISTOTLE***

THE INNER GAP

With high school behind me, I figured that I would no longer have to deal with having to fit in and people thinking they had the right to label me. I was wrong.

My struggle to gain confidence and become comfortable in my own skin continued as I entered adulthood. I was still afraid to be myself and worried I wouldn't fit in or be accepted because for so long, the messages I had heard were negative and discouraging. It seemed that no matter what I did, I wasn't good enough and along the way, I had accepted that 'fact' as my reality.

So, who did I have to be for the world to accept me as me? As you've heard through my story, finding myself was a windy road of highs and lows, learning and unlearning. As difficult as the journey was, it taught me a great deal about myself and enabled me to come to terms with my deep insecurities.

Over time, I learnt that most of us are living with unresolved emotions from our childhoods and we're uncomfortable in our own skins because we're focused on trying to fix the 'outside'. We focus on external things and overlook our internal environments. We try desperately to fix the outside instead of the inner void within.

It's common to see many people use external things—a new house, car, partner or job to 'fix' the hole inside. Now there's nothing wrong with having success and material possessions but using them to heal your emotional scars rarely works. On the other-hand, some people numb their inner void through things like, alcohol, gambling, drugs, or addictions like shopping and sex. Others use things like money or prestige to soothe and cover-up their innate insecurities.

The more we try to fix the external aspects of ourselves or see ourselves as internally broken, the less satisfied we feel inside because it means we are still not truly at peace with ourselves. Being at peace with yourself is the ultimate place to be. It enables you to stop striving for something to validate your worth and begin to feel worthy just because you exist. Living unashamedly as yourself brings a level of inner peace that nothing external can do.

If we live incongruently or in conflict with our core values, we tend to experience a lot of unrest and frustration. We continue to strive and never arrive.

In order to live peacefully within, we must stop living up to other people's expectations and start to live up to our own. We must cease to stop impressing others and start living joyfully within ourselves.

A way that I have found incredibly helpful in order to do this, is by embracing my vulnerability. It can be a scary thing to consider at first but believe me, it opens you up to new and exciting possibilities within yourself.

> *"BEAUTY IS BEING COMFORTABLE AND CONFIDENT IN YOUR OWN SKIN."*
> **IMAN**

EMBRACING VULNERABILITY

Showing people your vulnerability and weakness and strengths is part of showing who you actually are and allowing people to connect with you. I had to learn that. As author Madeleine L'Engle also noted, "When we were children, we used to think that when we were grown-up we would no longer be vulnerable. But to grow up is to accept vulnerability…To be alive is to be vulnerable."

Over the years, I have really wanted people to see on the outside how I felt on the inside. Although I've wanted to share my vulnerability, I was really afraid people would think of me as a fraud and that I had to present myself as someone who was strong and successful because I thought that was a part of being successful.

Sharing your struggles with other people is valuable because then people are able to relate to you. If people see you as a stoic invincible warrior, it can be hard for them to get past that and connect with you.

Vulnerability is an interesting state of being and often misunderstood. Many people associate vulnerability with being weak and emotionally fragile. We may have also been taught as children not to show vulnerability. Little boys are often told to "be a man," or "stop sooking".

With vulnerability also comes the possibility of rejection or failure so we try to avoid vulnerability as much as possible. But this is a trap. Being vulnerable is to be human. It's what makes us human. It's what connects us. Vulnerability is an important part of the human experience and can represent strength and courage rather than a weakness. Being vulnerable can actually help us work through and deal with our emotions, rather than pushing them away and burying them deep inside.

Bestselling author and researcher, Dr Brené Brown, an expert on social connection has carried out extensive research to discover what lies at the root of social connection and came to the conclusion that it is vulnerability.

According to Dr Brown, vulnerability encourages us to be honest and kind with ourselves and "is the core, the heart, the centre of meaningful human experiences. What makes you vulnerable makes you beautiful."[1]

Even though showing vulnerability can be uncomfortable, there are many benefits that come with embracing this part of ourselves:

- Vulnerability allows us to be totally honest and our authentic selves, rather than a watered-down version of who we are and trying to please other people.
- When we demonstrate vulnerability, we build empathy with others and encourage them to do the same. This means we remove those barriers to communication and are able to share feelings more easily, forgive more easily and give and receive love.
- Being vulnerable can help us work through our emotions more

effectively which is ultimately positive for our mental well-being.

- Each time we demonstrate vulnerability we become more resilient and courageous. This is because we push through fear and embrace what we are actually feeling and our true self.
- If you try and avoid vulnerability you are actually missing out on a very important part of life. For example, if you avoid trying something new, or embarking on a new relationship because you're afraid of failing or getting hurt, you're potentially missing out on life-changing experiences.

Now don't be me wrong, I'm not saying that embracing vulnerability is easy, it can feel very uncomfortable at first. But I am saying that if you start to peel off your layers and embrace your more vulnerable aspects, then you will become a more resilient, loving and authentic person.

THE ART OF FAILING FORWARD

"FAIL EARLY, FAIL OFTEN, BUT ALWAYS FAIL FORWARD."
JOHN C. MAXWELL

For me, an important part of vulnerability is feeling comfortable to admit when I've made a mistake.

We often hold ourselves back from making mistakes because of a fear of getting it wrong. But the only way to get over that is to make more mistakes. You can't grow and you can't get to where you want to be without a willingness to fail. I know that may make you squirm, who wants to make more mistakes, right? But part of embracing vulnerability is a willingness to show the imperfect side of yourself. We all have those aspects that are still under development so it's perfectly normal to have those areas. Being human means that you still have some aspects in life that you're wrestling with or slowly navigating through and working out in your own time. None of us are ten-foot tall and non-penetrable. That's just totally unrealistic.

For example, when I'm coaching, I explain to my clients that setting up and growing a business isn't pretty. I warn them that they're going to get dirty and bumped and that they'll make loads of mistakes along the way. Making mistakes is part of the process.

I think people need to hear this because there's a misconception out there of what success is and people need to understand that true growth is uncomfortable and messy. Through chaos comes new order. Think of the caterpillar, it goes through enormous change to morph and transform into the full beauty of a butterfly. Buddhist teacher, Thich Nhat Hanh had a saying—"No mud, no lotus." He said, "Most people are afraid of suffering. But suffering is a kind of mud to help the lotus flower of happiness grow. There can be no lotus flower without the mud."

From my experience, he's right. The pain can bloom the pinnacle. That's why I recommend people to use failing as a stepping stone to success. To view it as part of the journey.

One of my favourite books, *The Confidence Code* by authors and journalists, Katty Kay and Claire Shipman, looks at the psychology behind confidence—they ask: where it comes from, how to build it and why women seem to have less of it compared to men.[2] One of the key messages I've taken from this book and passed on to my clients is "to fail fast." That means to get out of your comfort zone and try lots of different ideas, expecting most of them will fail. Get comfortable with failure so it doesn't plague you and represent something that scares the pants off you. Risk-taking is vital for building confidence and you should act, even if you feel uncertain. Even just for practice.

To take risks of course takes a certain amount of courage but as author Anne Dillard reminded us, "You can't test courage cautiously."

How to fail fast:
- Don't overthink
- Act
- Be authentic

EMOTIONAL TERRITORY

Life is not just about success and failure, it involves so many other experiences. Sadly, losing people and things we love is obviously a part of living and it's important to allow yourself the space to grieve and not feel as though you have to push through or apologise for your emotions.

If you lose a loved one, or your business or job, grief is the normal response and how long you choose to stay there is your choice. Emotions are part of the human landscape and from a young age, many of us were taught that strong emotions were wrong and to be avoided. We were told not to show anger, or pride or sometimes even affection. As a result, many tend to have an embarrassment or fear around showing emotions.

When I was growing up, if you were upset about something people hated seeing this, so you were only given the space of about five seconds to experience this emotion.

Expressing raw emotion such as grief can still make many people feel uncomfortable even though it's a natural and normal part of life. No one is immune to grief and sadly we all lose loved ones. Avoiding emotions or numbing our feelings is a short-term 'solution' and not the answer to long-term emotional health and stability.

In life, we experience a huge array of emotions and it's important that we validate them and acknowledge them. Some studies show that repressing our emotions can lead to increased stress and disease. [3]

Having emotions whether "good" or "bad" is as natural as having sunshine and rain. They are both essential ingredients to life. Accepting the fact you will always have a flux of different emotions is a vital part of staying emotionally healthy. Learning how to express your emotional side is an important communication tool and something I explore with my clients.

I often remind them that feeling comfortable in their own skin and with their emotions is a continual process. And if they believe they're fully evolved and have arrived, then they're doomed for failure because life will always serve up a whole new set of challenges.

And that's the juicy part of life, it's totally unpredictable! If you believe that you have it all worked out and nothing can challenge you, then maybe it's time to head out of your comfort zone.

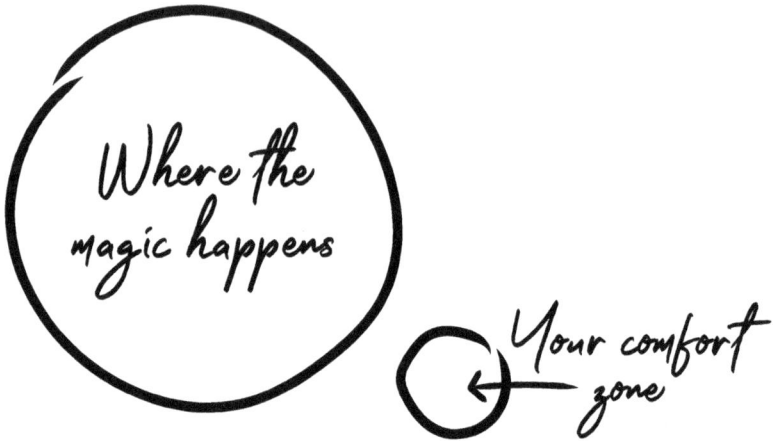

Where the
magic happens

Your comfort
zone

That attitude might work if you're content to rest on your laurels and not do anything more in your life. However, if you choose to leave your comfort zone, life will continue to challenge you.

If you want to achieve a new goal, it's going to require you to go through some messy moments and venture into new uncharted territory. Because let's be honest, if you're going into new territory there is going to be a certain amount of uncertainty and risk involved. I assume this is why Helen Keller said, "Life is a daring adventure or it's nothing." But that's what makes life exciting and the rewards worth it.

"

YOU CAN NEVER
CROSS THE
OCEAN UNTIL
YOU HAVE
THE COURAGE
TO LOSE SIGHT
OF THE SHORE.

"

André Gide

LOSING YOURSELF, FINDING YOURSELF

I had a client, Karen, who came to me for help after leaving an abusive marriage. She felt she had lost her identity and needed to reclaim her new sense of self.

Karen felt she couldn't speak her 'truth' anymore and basically felt lost. She was looking for a way to find her true self and express that in a meaningful way.

In working with Karen, I encouraged her to not feel ashamed of her experience and own her story—to see it as part of her life story. I encouraged her to talk about her experiences openly and honestly.

Sharing her story has allowed Karen to connect more authentically with others and let go of people's judgement and expectations of her. Part of this acceptance was being proud of the fact she had achieved financial independence outside her relationship and had done this on her own. The other aspect was the way she saw herself—she no longer saw herself as a victim but as a self-made woman. This identity shift was incredible. Karen accepted her past but didn't let it limit her. She accepted her life journey with all of its peaks and troughs and reclaimed her new chapter as an empowered self-made woman.

"You can always find the sun within yourself if you will only search."
Maxwell Maltz

UNLEASHING YOUR FIRST SUPERPOWER

FINDING THE OKAY SPACE INSIDE

We all need to find our own okay space inside, and the journey will be different for each and every one of us. Finding your own sense of self is a superpower! It fills you up with strength and helps you find your own innate wisdom and peace of mind.

In finding your okay space, I encourage you to engage in a three-step process: Reflect, Decide and Act.

REFLECT

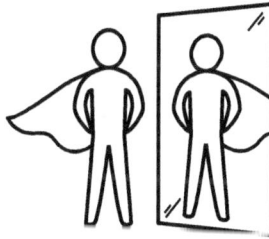

Growing up, what sort of child were you? Describe yourself in detail.

....

....

....

....

....

....

....

....

....

....

....

....

....

....

How were you perceived and described by others, especially adults? What labels were you given and have those 'labels' stayed with you?

....

....

....

....

....

....

....

....

....

....

....

Look over the labels you were given and write down how those labels have influenced your life and how you see yourself today?

....

....

....

....

....

....

....

....

....

....

....

Create new authentic and empowering labels for yourself—ones that feel true for you. Have you moved from victim to victor? Are you self-made, financially independent, emotionally intelligent?

....

....

....

....

....

....

....

....

....

....

....

....

....

....

....

DECIDE

To stop apologising for being your true self. Make a pact with yourself to cease apologising for being you. Be yourself on purpose.

To stop looking for validation from others.

To see your mistakes as an opportunity to learn and grow, rather than as representing failure.

To challenge people when they seek to invalidate your core traits.

ACT

Write down the qualities about yourself you are proud of. Don't hold back.

Looking back over your life—we all have things that have not worked out or gone our way. When you identify those areas—what could you take responsibility for in the outcome of those? What have you learnt from them that can help you move forward in your life? How can those experiences benefit you in the future?

Write down some compliments you have received from other people that have made an impression.

....

....

....

....

....

....

....

....

Recognising your new positive labels, what do they mean to you now? How can you express those labels more in the world?

....

....

....

....

....

....

....

....

Write a new life story to match your new labels. Who are you now with these new labels or identities?

"

TO BE COMFORTABLE IN YOUR OWN SKIN IS THE BEGINNING OF STRENGTH.

"

Charles Hendy

SUPERPOWER #2

Embracing Your Femininity

"

THINK LIKE
A QUEEN.
A QUEEN IS NOT
AFRAID TO FAIL.
FAILURE IS ANOTHER
STEPPING STONE
TO GREATNESS.

"

Oprah Winfrey

Purpose

Your femininity is a gift—embrace this
gift and learn to express it in all that
you do. When you deny any part of
yourself you will be out of balance and
alignment. Let us go on the journey
of self-acceptance and bring that
alignment back into your life.

Check out Alison's personal video to
you, the reader, about Superpower 2
in the bonus interactive book. Go to
deanpublishing.com/alisonwheeler
to discover more.

"

YOU ARE MANY TO MANY.
PEACEMAKER AND WAR
FIGHTER, SUPPLICANT,
ASPIRANT, PENITENT,
THE TRUE FRIEND,
THE TRUSTED SOUL,
THE TRUTH SPEAKER
AND YOU HAVE
BEEN DECEIVED.
BECAUSE NO MATTER
HOW SMALL AN ACT
OF KINDNESS OR
GENEROSITY OR
SIMPLY THE POSITIVITY
YOU PUT OUT IN THE
WORLD, IT WILL MAKE
A DIFFERENCE.[1]

"

Wonder Woman

Turning forty was an important turning point for me in many ways. I was happily married with a beautiful daughter and took pride in the success I had achieved over the years. Yet for some reason, I wasn't completely fulfilled and felt there was something missing on some level.

I found myself questioning why I continued to feel dissatisfied. Why was I continually chasing the next thing, after the next thing, yet it still wasn't enough? I love the game of success but something else was just not in alignment. I couldn't quite pinpoint what that something was but it was gnawing at me.

It was during this time that I began to realise there were parts of me that were really underdeveloped and that I really didn't understand.

Perhaps the most integral part of me—the part that I really didn't understand and had neglected for so long, was my feminine side.

I now understood my drive to succeed, at all costs, was the masculine way of doing things, but it wasn't leading to fulfilment.

Sure. It led to a lot of rewards, trophies and other recognition. I had reached national level in my rowing and bodybuilding, and achieving more than most could dream of. Yet, I always felt there was something missing.

I could see I wasn't really connected to myself, or to other people, because I was just chasing the next rabbit, and then the next one.

Reaching the age of forty, it dawned on me I knew nothing or little about being feminine—basic things like doing my hair nicely and putting on makeup. I wondered where and how women learnt this because I felt like I'd missed the boat on that part of being female.

Although getting my hair and nails done is not really a priority for me, I did question why I had no clue about these physical representations of femininity.

More importantly, I began to wonder what I may be missing on the inside, spiritually? This led me to think about what I was reflecting outwardly and how I was representing myself to other people.

And so began another process of peeling back the layers and examining myself. I critiqued how I was representing myself to the world and wondered whether maybe I was hiding under a different veil—a masculine veil.

I became more aware of how people were responding to me and the judgements they were making about my personality.

They would often make comments about my personality, saying things like "you're harsh," or "you have no feelings," "why do you have to be so driven?" I found these comments quite confusing and confronting because this was the way I had grown up—this was me.

Despite the judgements from people around me, I continued to strive, chasing those rabbits and then falling in a heap. The physical and emotional effects on my body were extreme—chronic fatigue, injuries, burnout—and it seemed to be an ongoing cycle.

Often, I wouldn't recognise the signs until it was too late. That was when I realised my body was trying to tell me something. It was desperately trying to communicate something important.

When I reached the age of forty, I thought—*is this how the rest of my life is going to be like?* I realised I needed to begin nurturing myself and end this pattern of destructive behaviour.

RESTORING BALANCE

Not surprisingly, statistics show that stress and burnout are affecting more women than men.[2]

I believe this is because women, today, are trying to succeed in a very and at everything all at once masculine way and trying to do everything all at once. This behaviour creates imbalance and often leads to mental fatigue, depression and a lack of true fulfilment.

As women, I believe we need to bring back a sense of balance and reconnect to our femininity. This means women need to be encouraged to return to the 'feminine' way of doing things, compared to the masculine way which is traditionally focused on dominance and winning at all costs.

For me, coming to this realisation was actually pretty amazing and represented a major turning point in my life. It was almost as if I was being handed an excuse to get out of that perpetual cycle of constantly driving myself to the point of exhaustion.

I realised, then, that I had to create an environment within myself where I felt safe to be feminine. This meant I had to think about the conversations I was having with the people in my life.

I had to be willing to confront certain things and communicate my concerns to them, rather than waiting until I fell over in a heap of exhaustion.

This meant learning to communicate more effectively and honestly. Once I felt safe in this new environment I had created, I would be able to express my needs and start nurturing my feminine side more.

It meant being able to tell my husband when I was feeling overwhelmed and not coping. It was about allowing him to challenge me when he thought I was taking on too much. Now I must admit, asking for help was a new and difficult thing for me to learn at first. It was about accepting and tapping into my feminine energy, learning to have a new relationship with my feminine side. I had to find, nurture and balance *my whole self*—both masculine and feminine parts.

FEMININE ENERGY

What is feminine energy and what does it really mean?

I believe it goes deeper than make-up and pretty clothes. It is far more complex and, to a certain extent, goes to the very heart of the human condition.

Different religions and cultures refer to feminine energy in different ways and have special symbols representing it, often a combination of feminine and masculine traits.

In Taoism, feminine energy is referred to as yin. Interestingly, according to Eastern philosophy, yin is one of two opposing energies, the other being yang, whose interaction is thought to influence everything in the universe. Yin is negative, dark and feminine, whereas yang is positive, bright and masculine.

In Hinduism, the Goddess Shakti is considered a divine cosmic energy, representing feminine energy, fertility and the dynamic forces that move through the universe. She is responsible for creation, an agent of change and a force that restores balance.

In ancient European cultures, Artemis was worshipped as the goddess of the hunt, the moon and chastity. In time, she also became associated with childbirth and nature.

Regardless of gender, we all have a combination of feminine and masculine energy. The balance between the two determines how we see the world and how we respond to it. This energy defines who we are.

Feminine energy is a very powerful force that is associated with traits such as creativity, connection, empathy, intuition, nurturing and vulnerability. Your feminine side is expressed when you move with the flow of life and embrace your creativity energy.

On the other hand, your masculine may express itself when you're working towards a goal, getting things done and driving forward.

I believe people can, and often do, have a combination of all these traits. None are inherent to any gender, but rather, describe two different and opposing ways of being.

Ideally, it's good for us to have outlets for both our masculine and feminine energies. However, in western culture masculine qualities tend to be valued more than feminine energy. When we over value masculine energy, we spend most of our time working and very little time resting and connecting with others.

Valuing female energy means prioritising down time—taking the time to create, to read, do yoga and simply enjoy the moment and regaining the balance we all need.

However, it's also important to remember that being feminine is not just about being quiet and rejuvenating. Feminine energy is also about being bold and courageous. It is the force of creativity and transformation which is a vital part of everyone.

If you feel burned out, overworked, fragmented or exhausted you need to call upon find your feminine energy to restore, inspire and enliven yourself.

"The union of feminine and masculine energies within the individual is the basis of all creation."

Shakti Gawain

EMBRACING YOUR FEMININITY

Consider the following traits. How many relate to you? Is there an imbalance within you?

Masculine Traits	Feminine Traits
Dominant	Trustworthy
Aggressive	Considerate
Competitive	Giving
Assertive	Flexible
Driven	Passionate
Direct	Diplomatic
Confident	Generous
Independent	Collaborative
Analytical	Authentic
Strong	Intuitive

MASCULINE	FEMININE
Rational	Perceptive
Confident	Thoughtful
Focused	Nurturing
Stable	Innovative
Reliable	Collaborative
Definitive	Sympathetic
Decisive	Responsive
Goal Driven	Grateful

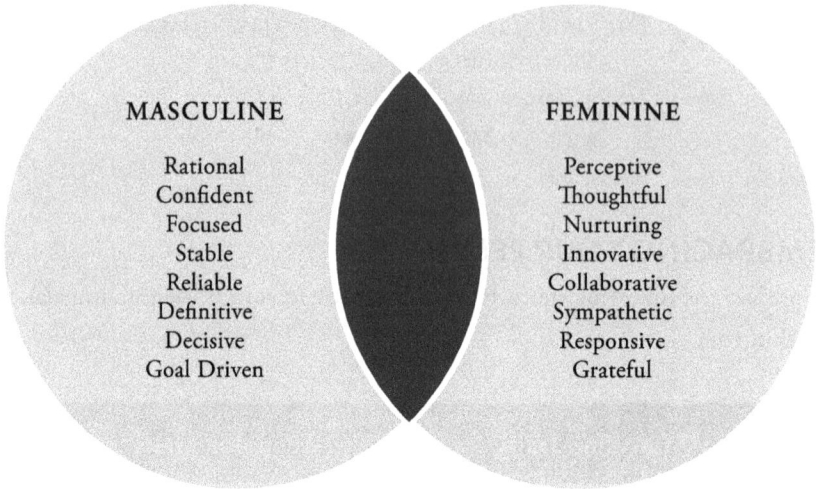

In their book *The Athena Doctrine*, authors John Gerzema and Michael D'Antonio, describe an emerging trend where people from several countries, from the United States to Korea, claimed to associate happiness, leadership, success and morality to the dominance of feminine traits.[3] The traits mentioned include nurturing and empathy, as well as collaboration, kindness, reliability and generosity.

I believe so many women are living with unempowered feminine energy and are overcompensating with masculine energy.

I know for myself, living a more authentic life and feeling more comfortable in the skin I have been given, means understanding and accepting my feminine energy.

But, how do you actually do this in your day to day life? I think many opportunities present themselves to us in our personal and work lives, but often we fail to pick up on them, missing these key opportunities.

SLOW DOWN

These days we live our lives at such a frantic pace there is little time to slow down and draw breath to stop and smell the roses that are all around us. You need time, space and solitude to identify and tap into your feminine power, so find some time in your day to deliberately slow down.

Perhaps step outside into nature, go for a walk, listen to some calming music, meditate. Spend time at a slower pace in order to nourish yourself. The frantic pace of life creates stress and stress brings premature ageing, hormone imbalances, chronic fatigue and anxiety. As American comedian and performer Eddie Cantor said, "Slow down and enjoy life. It's not only the scenery you miss by going too fast—you also miss the sense of where you are going and why."

I totally agree. If we give ourselves time to slow down and enjoy life, it gives us time to self-reflect and ensure we are connected with our values, our why, our goals and dreams. Slowing down means we don't get caught up in the crazy pace of life and lose ourselves in the doing, the chaos and the constant demands life throws at us.

For driven people like me, slowing down can be a discipline at first, you need to practice it. It doesn't always come naturally; but when you realise that it helps you stay in touch with your feminine energy, it can help you regenerate and revive you. It can be a form of self-care and mind therapy. Try and catch yourself when you get stuck in the frenzy of life and adjust yourself to slow down; slow down your actions and even your speech and movement until you rebalance yourself.

TUNE IN

Once you have taken a moment to slow down you now need to make a conscious effort to tune in to your feminine energy and listen to what your soul is telling you. To a certain extent, this is all about listening to what your intuitive side is telling you which is the very heart of feminine power.

Tuning in to your intuition is different for everybody, it often involves listening to your hunches, gut instincts or inner voice in a way that is subtle and sacred. It's learning to communicate with a deeper part of you that is connected to the universal intelligence; the part of you that knows rather than thinks.

Women in particular are naturally wired to their intuition. It's one of our superpowers and helps us connect, empathise and understand others at a level that isn't always communicated verbally. Intuition isn't something you only use in crisis, your intuition is within you and can be used in all situations; for example, in parenthood, at work, or even in sports.

Marilyn Monroe said, "A woman knows by **intuition**, or instinct, what is best for herself." And that is true. There is a deep instinct within our bodies that silently nudges us to do or say certain things despite logic.

However intuition is not only a female thing. We all have it. In fact, some of the most logical, practical and 'no nonsense' type masculine people, tap into the power of their intuition. Like Steve Jobs the mastermind of Apple. He advised people to—"Have the courage to follow your heart and **intuition**. They somehow already know what you truly want to become. Everything else is secondary." Albert Einstein called the intuition "a sacred gift", and "the father of supercomputing" Seymour Cray said, "I'm supposed to be a scientific person but I use **intuition** more than logic in making basic decisions."

Intuition is more than a feeling, it's deep guidance and worth learning to listen to.

Tuning into your mind, body and spirit allows you to tap into new and undiscovered resources you may be unacquainted with. If you have an underdeveloped feminine side, then quite possibly you've been blocking or suppressing your intuitive self. If so, take time to explore this part of yourself, take your internal nudges or hunches more seriously and give yourself time and space to listen to the intuitive beauty within.

IDENTIFY YOUR POWER SOURCE

Think about how you're reflecting yourself to others and where you're drawing your energy from. As we have both feminine and male traits within us, it's important to identify where your source of power is coming from. For example, for much of my life I was drawing my power from purely masculine energy sources—only relying on my drive and ambition to accomplish a goal. I was neglecting many feminine power sources such as intuition and relaxation. Hence, I was stuck in a vicious cycle of injury burnout and self-neglect. It's important to identify where you draw your power from so you can identify any major imbalances. You can start by identifying your primary power sources and any recurring patterns that you have.

For example, if you are considered "too blunt" or "too direct" and this is causing problems in your relationships,—then perhaps you could engage in some more diplomatic (feminine) behaviour and see if this generates a better result. Remember, balancing the masculine and feminine within yourself is true power. When our energies are out of balance (heavily masculine or heavily feminine) we then also find ourselves in imbalanced situations and relationships, or have imbalances within ourselves.

When you become self-aware and discover where you derive your power from, you then gain control of yourself and the situations you find yourself in. A good way to understand where you derive your power source from is through the mirror of others. You can ask yourself—*what part of myself am I representing to people? Am I being authentic or am I acting in a way that is merely expected of me in this particular situation?*

Think about the repetitive comments people have said and question if they are pointing to an imbalanced energy within you?

Sometimes we have different power sources for different situations. For example, one client I had was overly masculine in the workplace (direct, assertive, competitive) but she was the opposite in her relationship (needy, insecure and indecisive). She swayed rapidly in her energy depending on the situation and needed to learn new skills to balance them both. She could retain her power in both areas of her life but she would benefit from enhancing the polarity of the energy she was lacking in.

Being self-aware of your power source for your primary areas in life is very helpful to you as it enables you to have greater harmony and fulfilment in all areas of your life. It's not about 'being wrong', it's about harmony within and being able to enjoy the best of both worlds.

CHOOSE THE TRAITS YOU NEED

Once you have tapped into your feminine side and identified the origins of your energy, it's important to choose what traits you need to harness to serve you best. Perhaps it's time to tap into those powerful feminine traits like vulnerability, compassion, empathy and creativity that you have kept buried? Or perhaps you are a walkover and being continually taken advantage of and need more masculine traits in certain situations?

Society has leaned towards empowering the masculine traits in many areas of life and suffocated or suppressed the feminine. It's important to not just go with what society expects but to really nurture what helps you be your best. For me, I needed to develop my feminine side and explore my vulnerability. I needed to keep my drive (masculine) but not let it drive me into further burnout. Embracing my feminine energy not only saved me from further self-destruction but it allowed me to nourish myself inside and out.

Others may need just to tweak aspects of their life rather than do a massive overhaul and develop severely underdeveloped aspects of self. It all begins with awareness.

Ask yourself—*where do I need to tweak the balance? What would serve me most in this situation?*

TAME YOUR INNER CRITIC

Be aware of the 'stories' you tell yourself and of negative self-talk. Perhaps you question whether it's acceptable to show your vulnerability, or if you're being too nice and that people are going to walk all over you? Start to challenge and reframe the stories that disempower you and celebrate your vulnerability.

Maybe you were taught not to show weakness or not to express yourself. Maybe you grew up with messages that suppressed your uniqueness, or made it wrong. Challenging those old identities can help free you from their boundaries.

One of the first things you can do is stop criticising yourself. Stop berating your weak points. Stop rejecting compliments and deflecting kind offers or gestures from others. Embrace yourself in a new way. Often that means, taming your inner critic. You know the one I mean. The voice that tells you—*you can't*—and lists all the reasons why you can't regardless of their validity. Some people's inner critic gets too much stage time. It's demanding and relentless and can also be blaming and shaming.

It can say things like—*you're not good enough*! That could mean that you're not smart enough, brave enough, talented enough, tall enough, skinny enough, funny enough, confident enough …or whatever other words you want to add.

Your inner critic is just that—a critic! It loves criticism. It thrives in it; and there's only one way to tame it. Stop feeding it with more criticism. You probably can't eradicate it (as we all still have that pesky little voice inside)—but you can quiet it down and tame it into submission. You start by talking to yourself in a different way, in a kinder way, a more encouraging way. You cease the critiques! And start feeding yourself with empowering inner talk. This reduces the stage time given to your inner critic. As author Alan Cohen said, "If you gave your inner genius as much credence as your inner critic, you would be light years ahead of where you now stand."

It's time to tame your inner critic and let your inner genius shine bright.

NURTURE YOURSELF

A simple and enjoyable way to honour your feminine side is to nurture yourself with special treats such as soaking in a long bath, filling your home with flowers or taking care of your wellbeing.

If self-care isn't something you're used to doing or are familiar with, then don't worry—I have made you a list of awesome ways you can love and nurture your wellbeing.

- Have a long bath or spa
- Take a walk in nature
- Listen to a guided meditation
- Binge watch your favourite show
- Go out for coffee with a good friend
- Get your nails done
- Fill your home with flowers
- Light candles and dim the lights and put your feet up and rest
- Put your favourite music on
- Listen to podcasts or YouTube clips that promote self-care

- Take a break from social media
- Read a book
- Cuddle with your pets
- Garden or plant some veggies
- Go out into the sun and have a picnic
- Get a massage
- Indulge in something creative that you enjoy
- Go shopping and buy something only for you
- Get your hair done or have a facial
- Nourish yourself with a nutritious meal
- Do Yoga or mindfulness
- Make a vision board
- Take a nap

*"IF YOU FEEL 'BURNOUT' SETTING IN, IF YOU FEEL
DEMORALIZED AND EXHAUSTED, IT IS BEST, FOR
THE SAKE OF EVERYONE, TO WITHDRAW AND
RESTORE YOURSELF. THE POINT IS TO HAVE
A LONG-TERM PERSPECTIVE."*

DALAI LAMA

SPEAK YOUR TRUTH

Speaking truth, combined with kindness, is a key part of your feminine energy and not something you need to apologise for. In life, we need to define ourselves before we allow others to do it for us. As Audre Lorde, self-described "black, lesbian, mother, warrior, poet," said "If I didn't define myself for myself, I would be crunched into other people's fantasies for me and eaten alive."

Speaking your truth doesn't have to be a raw, in-your-face style like Audre's (but it can be too). Speaking your truth is really about being authentic, being open and honest with who you are and controlling your own narrative.

When I speak my truth, I am honouring a relationship I have with myself. I am staying true to my values and communicating that to others. When you speak your truth, you don't have to do it standing on a stage yelling "your truth" to the masses. It's much more humble than that. It's staying true to your values every day and not being afraid to be you. It's sometimes staying 'no' when society pressures you to say 'yes'. It sometimes saying 'yes' when others pressure you to say 'no'. It's about speaking up if you see something you don't agree with or sitting down when you feel not sharing is better.

The point is—it's your choice. You get to choose who you share your truth with and who you don't.

In life, there will always be communication breakdowns or hard conversations that arise, mastering the skill of speaking your truth in a calm and considerate way is an incredible skill to have in your toolkit. This way of communicating combines the feminine aspects of kindness, honesty and caring with the masculine aspect of directness. They balance each other in a way that promotes clear and effective communication without compromising your femininity. It enhances your feminine traits and allows you to be extra masterful in the way you share your truth. It gives you strength and softness simultaneously.

NURTURE YOUR RELATIONSHIPS

Think about the energy you harness when it comes to your relationships. Do you fall into the trap of being too controlling, needing to control and dominate, focusing too much of your masculine energy at the expense of your feminine side? Do you need to restore the balance in this part of your life?

Relationships are crucial to our happiness. We are social creatures and thrive in harmonious relationships. When our relationships aren't working well, we feel out of balance and unhappy.

Masculine and feminine energies are gender specific; they are embodied energies by both males and females. What creates that spark in intimate relationships is the polarity between the energies. Think of the polarity of a magnet—it has two distinct types of poles: positive and negative. They attract and repel and work together to form magnetism.

When the energy is too similar (no polarity) quite often there is no spark or magnetism between the two energies. Learning to recognise this and rebalance the energies in your relationship/s can completely transform them.

In relationships, feminine energy is: emotional, fluid, flexible, surrendering and permissible. Whereas the masculine energy is logical and directive and action-orientated. For example, when in conflict, the feminine energy seeks to communicate and connect to resolve the issues, whereas the masculine energy often seeks solitude and retreats in order to problem solve.

Learning to nurture and understand the polarity of energies within your relationship is a key to honouring them and savouring their exquisite differences. The more polarity—the greater the attraction.

I often recommend to my clients, to recognise the energies within themselves and to learn about masculine and feminine energies in relationships. There are some incredible books and teachers on this topic including Anthony Robbins, author of *The Five Love Languages*, Gary Chapman, and many others on YouTube.

> *"When both sexes rise to power, one cannot triumph over the other because neither is more powerful than the other. There will be balance."*[4]
>
> **Teal Swan**

BE CREATIVE

One of the most powerful and intuitive ways to tap into your feminine energy is by doing something creative, whether that's cooking, gardening, painting, craft, dancing, music—no matter what you're creating this is all about tapping into the creative soul we all have and allowing it to express itself.

In fact, current research shows that people who engage in creative activities have higher levels of happiness and wellbeing than those who have no creative pursuits.[5]

And furthermore, even simple acts of self-expression, for example, colouring-in or doodling show that our brains receive 'reward' signals and increase feelings of personal enjoyment.[6]

You don't need to consider yourself a creative person to enjoy creative pursuits, you can simply add 'creative thinking' into your current activities and explore new ways of doing things. For example, if you're a business owner, you could draw your future plan on a whiteboard or vision board and use colour and visuals you get your creative juices flowing. Or if you are cooking dinner, you could put some music on and get flamboyant with a new recipe while dancing to your favourite tune.

You can get creative by dressing in new colours or wearing a new shade of lipstick. You can ignite your creativity with new experiences like painting, dancing, life-drawing, scrapbooking, pottery (just think of the movie *Ghost* if you think pottery is boring—it will change your mind).

I get a lot of creative enjoyment through cooking, exploring new cafes or wandering through organic health food stores. I also get a lot of creative inspiration from long walks on the beach or indulging in some Bikram Yoga. These types of activities automatically switch me into my feminine energy and allow my intuition, creativity and natural ease to rise to the fore.

MY CLIENT'S STORY

I had one client who came to me seeking help because, like me, she had reached burnout. She was a high level, driven athlete, career woman, wife and mother—trying to do it all and be all things to all people. She was not taking any time out for self-care and burning the candle at both ends.

In fact, she reminded me a lot of myself!

As we worked together, I encouraged her to reflect on her life and attitudes, suggesting that she was perhaps out of balance and alignment and needed to look at her process for achieving success. What was missing? What was leading to burn out? What had to change, and what was she willing to change? How could she be more authentic in her expression of success and embrace all of herself—both her feminine, as well as her masculine side?

After working with me, my client has gone on to be more in alignment—calmer, less hurried and, interestingly, more successful overall. She has changed her attitude from, *I will or must do it all,* to, *I can do it all but only with support and I chose what and when.*

Moving her attitude, moved her pressures. Realising that 'doing it all' was causing her to burnout, and burning out was causing her to feel exhausted, depleted and ignite feelings of failure. Her change of pace and attitude allowed her to move with more presence, more grace and enjoy her life rather than pile on more things 'to do'. She stopped piling up her to-do list and started to think of her 'to be' list. How could she be there for herself? How could she feel more relaxed and still accomplish her goals? How could she be more aligned and balanced?

Realising that she actually needed support was the small change she needed to make massive shifts in her life.

UNLEASHING YOUR SECOND SUPERPOWER
EMBRACING YOUR FEMININE ENERGY AND FINDING BALANCE

For so many of women, juggling careers, relationships and parenthood, life can be incredibly hectic, leaving us little time to take a step back and reevaluate how we're approaching life—the pressures we're putting on ourselves as we strive to compete in what continues to be a 'man's world.'

In order to tap into your feminine energy and restore some balance in your life, I encourage you to go through these questions:

REFLECT

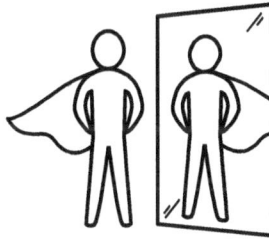

How do you feel at the end of the day? Calm and energised or tired and depleted? Are you using only masculine tendencies and need to balance them with more feminine ones?

....

....

....

....

....

....

How often do you seek validation from others? And what do you seek validation for? How often do you apologise? And to whom?

....

....

....

....

....

....

....

Can you identify the source of your energy in your work, home-life and relationships? Write a reflection.

....

....

....

....

....

....

....

....

DECIDE

To nurture yourself and make self-care a priority. What are some things you could do to begin this process? (I did a small list in this chapter to help you out.) Make your own personal list below and decide which one you will implement this week.

....

....

....

....

....

....

....

....

....

....

....

....

....

....

To speak the truth and be authentic, even when difficult conversations arise.

To ask for help and delegate tasks to others. What tasks could you delegate? Who could you ask for help? Or could you hire some help?

ACT

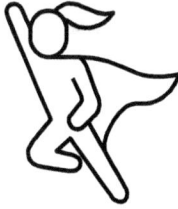

Find a creative outlet for yourself that reflects your unique spirit. Brainstorm a list here:

....

....

....

....

....

....

....

....

....

....

Fill your home with flowers.

Nourish your body with healthy food.

Tame that inner critic and stop the negative self-talk. Make a list of negative things you often say and replace them with positive statements.

Negative statements	Positive replacements
"I'm not good enough."	"You have all the tools you need to succeed."

The Gift of Self-Expression

"

BE YOURSELF;
EVERYONE ELSE IS
ALREADY TAKEN.

"

Oscar Wilde

Purpose

The purpose for this chapter is for
you to find your confidence and
courage and express it into the world
in your unique way.

There is no one like you, success for
you doesn't look like anyone else.

The world deserves to see you and have
your value added to everything you do.

BE YOU—we want to see that.

Check out Alison's personal video to
you, the reader, about Superpower 3 in
the bonus interactive book. Go to
deanpublishing.com/alisonwheeler
to discover more.

"

OUR DEEPEST FEAR
IS NOT THAT WE
ARE INADEQUATE.
OUR DEEPEST
FEAR IS THAT WE
ARE POWERFUL
BEYOND MEASURE.

"

Marianne Williamson

Throughout my own journey of self-development, I have come to the conclusion that we are all here on this planet with a specific gift.

We may not necessarily know what that gift is, but regardless of where we are on our journey, self-expression is the most important gift we have been given and we should use it.

I believe that if you're not fully expressing who you are to the world, then there's an aspect of you that's suppressed and not being fulfilled. Being self-expressed means people will see your true spirit and character. They will see the totality of who you are.

We all express ourselves in different ways and it really doesn't matter how you choose to do so. It's more important that it feels right for you. It could be through sport, cooking, art, gardening—whatever makes you feel alive and fully connected to your true self. Whatever you feel displays your unique individuality, your true spirit and character.

Full self-expression often involves taking a leap of faith which can be scary but the gifts you'll receive in return will far outweigh the discomfort.

"Bring your whole self to the experience. Because the more we do that, the more that people get to see that, the more comfortable everybody's gonna be with it."
Bozoma Saint John

BUILDING MYSELF, SCULPTING MY EXPRESSION

When I moved from New Zealand to Western Australia after completing my Occupational Therapy Degree, I worked in the outback regional town of Kalgoorlie for a couple of years. It was during that time that my father was diagnosed with stage-4 cancer so I made the decision to move to Queensland so I could travel back and forth to New Zealand to see him more easily. I took on additional studies at James Cook University and ended up volunteering at an Olympic Weightlifting Gym in Brisbane and meeting my future husband Paul. As you know, we fell in love, had a beautiful daughter and the rest as they say, is history.

Motherhood didn't slow me down, but it did help me rearrange my priorities and add a new, incredible dimension to my life.

After becoming a mum, I continued in various sports—weightlifting, CrossFit and anything else that involved a challenge. I eventually hit the stage where my usual daily exercise, clean eating and regimented discipline wasn't hitting the sweet spot. I still felt like I was missing something. Like the way that I felt on the inside didn't exactly match the outside. All the work was not paying off. When I looked in the mirror, I wasn't totally happy with what I saw—my physique didn't match my efforts. I knew I needed a massive shake-up. To express myself in a new way and find new elements within me. For me, this wasn't totally how I looked—it was much more—it was also about how I felt on the inside, how I was seeing myself as a woman.

I wanted to be more self-expressed and go to the next level in my business, my health and my self-development.

Yes, I was competing and doing CrossFit at that stage, training 6 days a week, but my hormones were out of balance and fatigue and injury was setting in. I was training a lot but not looking or feeling how I wanted to. I wasn't feeling energised and vibrant despite my health regime.

As I turned 40, I decided I wanted to change. I noticed a friend had changed her physique and was looking so much happier, so I asked her about it. I went and saw her coach and worked with that coach for a while. The coach suggested that I needed a new goal and focus, and to stop doing things that were harming and draining me.

Over time, we tried a few different things—triathlon training amongst others. When she suggested bodybuilding, it sparked something within me and all the dots connected—something deep inside said *yes*.

This intuitive hit was all about my personal journey and unleashing the feminine energy within. And so my bodybuilding journey began.

I started to take this new sport seriously. I knew I had to focus on improving my health and wellbeing, and rebalance my crazy hormones.

Bodybuilding gave me the perfect way to express myself and become more connected to my spirit. Even though it really didn't make sense to anyone else but me, I knew it was the answer I had been seeking. (This was one of those breadcrumb ideas I mentioned in earlier chapters). I needed to move from burnout to breakthrough and transform myself inside and out. And to do that, I needed to do things differently! I believe when we ask for something—the universe gives us an opportunity.

Sometimes, at first glance it may not be what you expected, or even wanted—but after a while, it may be what you needed. That's what bodybuilding was for me. It fulfilled something inside and that shone on the outside.

Admittedly, I didn't know anything about the bodybuilding world when I began, but it was part of the broader sporting world—a world I'd been involved in since the age of five. A world I felt very comfortable in. So I knew I had to learn the ropes and be a beginner again.

This sport was outside my comfort zone and I knew it would challenge and confront me by bringing up all my issues about being a woman and the outrageous expectations held by society. For example, the stereotypical notions about what a woman should look like and the expectations around beauty, femininity and age.

As I went along on the bodybuilding journey, a part of me was thinking, *this is ridiculous, what am I doing?* I had to give up and change a lot of things in my life in order to follow through with this demanding discipline. But the more I trained and got into the sport, the more I loved it.

For so many years prior, I had pushed my body to extremes and suffered the consequences—injuries, glandular fever, an eating disorder that left me feeling weak and depleted. However, with bodybuilding, I felt strong again—that I was fully expressing myself through gaining strength and sculpting my body. It felt so good!

Although bodybuilding is incredibly physically demanding (some may even describe it as a form of self-punishment), I didn't see it that way because I expressed myself through it and it fit the vision I had for myself at the time. I was moulding my body and mind in a new way.

Because of that, I love the sport! I don't love every single aspect of it, because everything you do has parts that you don't like, but for me bodybuilding is about me nurturing myself and evolving as an individual.

I took the bodybuilding journey as a way to rediscover myself and match my inside-self with my outside-self. It worked. It was the ultimate transformation for me physically, mentally and emotionally.

> *"IT IS A SHAME FOR A WOMAN TO GROW OLD*
> *WITHOUT EVER SEEING THE STRENGTH AND*
> *BEAUTY OF WHICH HER BODY IS CAPABLE."*
> **SOCRATES**

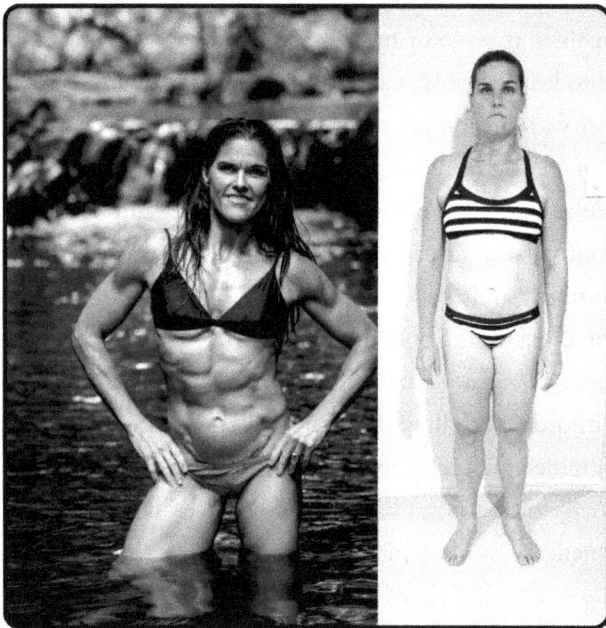

This is a photo of my personal transformation between 2018–2019

Right-hand side: this was me when I was training my ass off at CrossFit. I was eating well, following a strict diet and giving CrossFit my all. But something was missing for me.

Left-hand-side: this is me after 9 months of bodybuilding, injury-free and feeling strong and full of energy.

SELF-EXPRESSION IS UNIQUE

Each person's choice of self-expression is unique to them. I chose bodybuilding as my way of expressing myself, but for you, it may be something totally different—it may be art or fashion, sport or theatre.

It really doesn't matter how you choose to express yourself, just so long as it is something that brings you joy and fulfilment. I think choosing how we express ourselves goes somewhat deeper than simply choosing a hobby or signing up for a class.

Self-expression goes to the very core and essence of who you are and is an integral part of living an authentic life. As Coco Chanel said, "A girl should be two things: who and what she wants."

I also found that how you do one thing is how you do everything —wherever you go there you are. So as I became more expressed in bodybuilding and my physical body and feminine presence; I also noticed this flowed into other areas of my life: my business and personal relationships improved. Funny how that happens.

Looking back, I can clearly see the top five tips that helped me invigorate my self-expression and unleash my true self. I will share them below with you.

FIVE WAYS TO FULLY EXPRESS YOURSELF

1. Work out who you are

To be fully expressed it's important to step back from your life, reflecting on who you really are, rather than how people think you should be, and whether you are truly happy and fulfilled. Ask yourself what matters to you. Spend time writing down your values and what matters to you most. Who are you at your core?

Most people don't stop to ask themselves these deep questions. They instead spend their valuable time, chasing popularity, money and status and dismiss the inner pleading of their soul.

As Will Rogers famously said, "Too many people spend money they haven't earned, to buy things they don't want, to impress people that they don't like."

Now, we all need to pay bills and put food on the table, but we don't have to compromise ourselves to do it.

Working out who you are and being that person on purpose is part of your life's mission. It's deep and important work. It will change your life and you let it.

2. Speak truth and be authentic

Speaking openly and honestly is one of the best life skills you can have. Keeping your words aligned with your authentic self is part of the journey towards self-mastery. So often we wish we had been more honest and forthright when someone says or does something that hurts us. We often end up feeling disempowered and replaying the conversation or situation in our heads. Ultimately, not speaking honestly can affect our self-esteem and even our health.

In order to express yourself, try not to always avoid difficult conversations and confrontation. Your voice matters in a conversation and your opinion is equally as valid as someone else's. Speak the truth and make your words match your values.

One pioneering person who did this very thing was a woman named Margaret Kuhn. Margaret founded a movement called the Gray Panthers after she was forced to retire at the age of 65. Back then, in the USA, mandatory retirement was a law and people were forced to retire from work whether they liked it or not. Margaret opposed the idea of mandatory retirement and criticised ageist attitudes that society promoted. At the age of 65 she became an avid spokesperson for human rights and elderly rights; she formed a group of other passionate retirees and formed the Gray Panthers movement, a group dedicated to awareness about ageism in society and living vitally regardless of age. The group grew to over 40,000 members in her time. The reason I am telling you about Margaret is because she not only changed people's attitudes to age, but she spoke honestly and advocated for the need to speak things out loud. She famously said, "Leave safety behind. Put your body on the line. Stand before the people you fear and **speak your mind**—even if your voice shakes."

What great advice. *Speak your mind—even if your voice shakes.*

Notice she didn't say conquer the fear of speaking up. In fact, speaking your truth isn't always easy, but it's priceless in the fact it keeps your self-esteem and authenticity intact forever. Saying what you mean and meaning what you say can take a lot of practice, but it's truly an act of bravery.

3. Define yourself broadly and don't allow yourself to be labelled

We sometimes believe we are a certain way, with a fixed set of skills and strengths, and we live our life accordingly. For full self-expression we need to have the courage to recreate ourselves at any time and choose new ways of thinking and being. You may find you have talents and passions that never existed.

The term "fixed mindset" was originally coined by leading psychologist Dr Carol Dweck, an expert on human motivation. She noticed that some people believed their talents, strengths and intelligence were fixed; for example, if they weren't good at sports in their youth, they believed they were always going to struggle in that area and nothing could change that "fact".

She also noticed that there were people who believed that with effort and learning, they could improve over time; these people she described as having a "growth mindset". People who have a growth mindset also believe that setbacks are a normal part of the process and don't become discouraged if they have a few hiccups on the way.

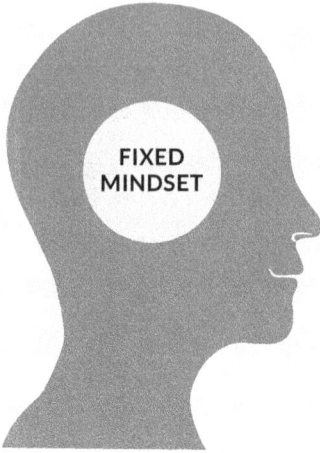

Fixed Mindset

"My intelligence is fixed and won't change."

"I am either good or natural at something or I'm not."

"I take criticism personally."

"It's difficult to improve."

"There's no point in even trying."

"I'm really not good at this."

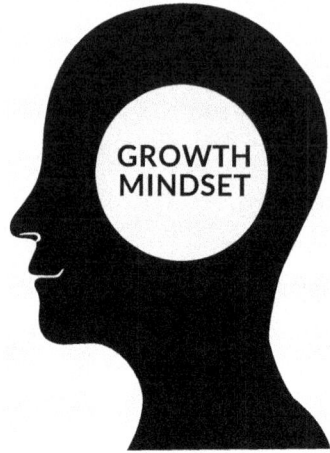

Growth Mindset

"I can improve if I keep trying."

"Other people's successes inspire me."

"Mistakes help me learn and grow."

"I learn a lot from challenges."

"Feedback is valuable and makes me better."

"I can learn anything if I put my mind to it."

Adapted from the work of Carol Dweck

Dweck's research discovered that people with a growth mindset can enjoy the benefits of—less depression and feeling of discouragement, reduced burnout and higher levels of motivation and personal satisfaction.[1]

So, it's important to not lock yourself into fixed ideas; to not grasp too tight to the way you believe you are, and instead give yourself room to try and enjoy new parts of yourself, or new hobbies. It's never too late to choose new ways to express yourself.

4. Pursue your passions and stop putting them on the backburner

Do you feel you're not fully expressing yourself to the outside world and ignoring those crazy ideas that pop into your head at times? If you don't pursue your passions, you'll end up not fulfilling your potential and with regrets.

Do you have anything you always wanted to do but just never took the time to make it happen? Perhaps life got in the way, or you got too busy, or you felt that moment had passed and you were now too old to try?

Take time to rekindle your passion. Pursue things that light you up. It doesn't mean that you have to do it for a living, it means you do things that ignite passion within you.

Your potential can only reach full maturity if you allow it to. Nourish yourself with the fertile soil so you can bloom into your best self.

5. Listen to your intuitive voice

Sometimes your inner voice knows what you need. Do you have a little voice inside calling for you to fulfil your potential?

Do you feel as though you are expressing yourself fully or is there something missing? Do you need to make some changes in your life?

Maybe your inner guide (your intuition) knows something deep within.

The word intuition is described as "the direct knowing or learning of something without the conscious use of reasoning," and "the ability to perceive or know things without conscious reasoning."[2]

Your intuition is different from your instinct and needs to be treated as such. Your intuition is more of an inner knowing whereas instinct is a reaction to an alert or sudden situation. Intuition doesn't use conscious reasoning, in fact it often bypasses logic and sends you hints, nudges and callings that you feel drawn to, or compelled towards. That's how bodybuilding felt for me, a little voice said yes despite the fact my brain could have easily said—*hell no*. I could feel something inside calling me and confirming that it was my next adventure.

Maybe your intuition has been calling to your next adventure? A signal from within to explore new parts of yourself or reinvent yourself in a way that fulfils your potential. Listen to that sacred voice within. Pay attention to its whispers—what is it calling you towards?

REKINDLING JOY—THE STORY OF A BALLERINA

One of my clients, Maggie, was a very high achiever—yet she felt unhappy and unfulfilled in her life. She had enjoyed a successful corporate career and, in her younger years, was a talented ballerina, performing at a national level. However, she left ballet behind after experiencing episodes of stage fright and feeling as though she had hit a wall with her dancing.

Later she also left her corporate career because she felt stifled and unhappy, even though she was still very successful.

When I began working with my client, we looked at her basic needs—was she getting enough sleep? Was she eating enough and properly hydrated?

Once we had sorted out her basic needs, we were able to move onto the ways she chose to express herself—focusing on her passions and those things in her life she found to be joyful.

Maggie admitted that although she had chosen to walk away from her ballet career, her love of dancing was still very much in her heart. In fact, she told me when she was not dancing, she felt unexpressed, less joyful and not as complete.

It was obvious that Maggie expressed herself through movement and dance, through the language of the arts and your unique expression of it. I asked her if she'd consider dancing again. Not necessarily for external achievement but to express herself fully.

With my encouragement, Maggie has since returned to dancing and is feeling the joy and fullness this beautiful artform is giving her. She said it's something she has not felt for a very long time.

Being able to truly express herself again, Maggie discovered that she had renewed energy and her vitality returned, which carried over into her business, resulting in a lot more success.

Maggie made room for her passion. She didn't decide to quit her day job and become a ballerina again. She understood that dance was the way she expressed herself, dance fulfilled something within her that only she could know. It gave her soul, life. It gave her back a part of herself that was dormant but needed to be expressed in order to feel vital.

> *"You are an artist of the spirit. Find yourself and express yourself in your own particular way."*
> **Don Miguel Ruiz**

CONNECTION, ADMIRATION AND GRATITUDE

I believe another very important aspect of self-expression is accepting there are different roles you can and will play throughout life. This will require you to choose how you respond to the inevitable ups and downs on the rollercoaster that is life.

You can be the angry, negative person who thinks nothing's going right for you. Or, you can dig deep and find something to admire and be grateful for. It's a choice.

I think it's really easy to find what's wrong with everything. Just take a look at current global events and it's very easy to feel overwhelmed and upset about all the things not going well. It's much more difficult to find what's right with things.

But to do this involves careful thinking about how you react and respond to the negative things that happen in your life. As the ancient saying from Epictetus goes, "It's not what happens to you but how you react to it." Attitude is everything. So picking one that will help propel you forward towards your vision is a smart move.

Let's not forget others either. Creating a life generally involves other people, especially if you're wanting an enriched and fulfilling one. Relationships are a huge part of our lives and a factor in our personal happiness. Connecting with others and communicating well are extremely important part of being able to achieve your goals and the vision you have for your life.

For example, my husband and I had a social media smear campaign directed against us, involving our business. The things being posted were terrible and some people believed the cruel things that were being said. We could have fought back and brought in the lawyers, but we chose to not go down that path. It was far better for us to communicate a more positive message to our followers and succeed at a higher level.

Your critics and haters actually want you to react angrily—they want a reaction. But if you play their game and get in the trenches beside them, you end up all muddy and bloody and it doesn't go anywhere.

Alternatively, you can just continue to play your own game and raise your own level of communication above the negativity of those who try to bring you down. Conflict can only survive when two participate. When one plays by themselves, it's not much of a game, right?

Now, I'm not saying this is an easy thing to do, but it's about going back to finding the okay space inside yourself—having the confidence to deal with the haters and the attackers. Looking back over my early life, especially to my school years, when I suffered so much bullying, I wish I'd known what I know now.

My haters at the time, did drag me into the trenches with them and, in response I retaliated by becoming a bully myself. I also responded by driving myself to exhaustion and punishing my body. I now know there is a better way. You raise your standards and refuse to stoop to the lower levels chosen by others. Taking the high road requires a lot of discipline and inner strength but it actually helps you stay out of the dirty games that negative people or trolls choose to play.

COMMUNICATING AT A HIGHER LEVEL

I remind my clients that life is not always going to be smooth sailing and there will be people who will actively set out to undermine and disempower you. As the saying goes, "haters are gonna hate". That's what they do, in fact, they excel at it.

If and when this happens to my clients, I always tell them that they need to revisit their vision. They need to cling to their values. I ask them—"Does your *ideal* life involve people like that?" They always say—"No, it doesn't." So why choose to engage with them? Don't! Hold tight to your vision when people want to knock you off your direction.

This can be a challenging thing to do because we're taught to engage the enemy and go to war against them. But once you're thinking about the 'war', you're no longer focused on your vision which means that you're being derailed and distracted from the vision you have created for yourself. When that happens. you need to dust yourself off, move on and get back on track with your life and your vision. Never allow the naysayers to control your vision. Only you do that.

In order to deal with critics and stick to your vision, it's important to learn how to communicate effectively and at a higher level.

Some of the most successful leaders of our time have achieved greatness because of their ability to communicate at the highest and most effective levels. Communication is possibly the most required trait when it comes to leadership and achieving your vision. It is also the most obvious sign of a person's emotional intelligence, the confidence they have in themselves and their ability to influence others.

Communication is an artform and skill—it can be learnt by anyone willing to improve at it. Communication can make or break our relationships. It can mend problems or make problems. It can harm or heal.

Learning the art of communication is now a business must! It's not enough to have a good product or a good service—you must be willing to communicate your message in a congruent and powerful way. You must be able to speak the language of the people in a way that is honest and transparent.

Recent data outlined by *Harvard Business Review* showed that the most important skill required *at any level* in business and leadership was communication.[3] It didn't matter if the job role was that of a CEO, junior employee or senior manager—communication was rated the most essential skill by over 330,000 people.

*"THE DIFFERENCE BETWEEN MERE MANAGEMENT AND
TRUE LEADERSHIP IS COMMUNICATION."*
SIR WINSTON CHURCHILL

So what does it take to be a great communicator? Here are my top 8 tips to mastering communication in your relationships.

TIPS FOR EFFECTIVE COMMUNICATION

1. Good communicators are also great listeners. Listen as you were going to repeat back the conversation. This is a very effective way to train yourself to focus on being an attentive listener.
2. Don't just listen—watch. A good communicator pays attention to both verbal and non-verbal communication such as body language and facial expressions.
3. Avoid the blame game rather inspire by your example operate from a place of curiosity and compassion instead of judgement.
4. Adapt your communication style to the person and the situation.
5. Show appreciation and gratitude in conversation. Appreciate other people's point of view (even if they are opposite to your own views) and show gratitude for the dialogue you are sharing.
6. Don't avoid difficult conversations. Use disagreements as an opportunity to see a different perspective, start a dialogue and find common ground.
7. Show empathy. This is a hallmark of emotional intelligence which means you are hearing the other person and can see the situation from their perspective.
8. Don't be afraid to apologise. Emotionally intelligent people are not afraid to admit when they are wrong and apologise in a sincere way.

UNLEASHING YOUR THIRD SUPERPOWER
FINDING YOUR SPECIAL GIFT OF EXPRESSION

REFLECT

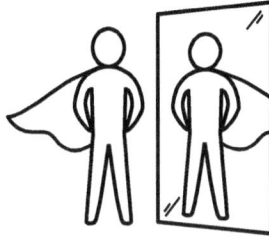

Do you sometimes have a sense there is a certain lack of joy and energy in your life? Why do you think that is?

....

....

....

....

....

....

....

....

....

....

....

....

What did you love doing as a child? When was the last time you did this?

Do you have something in your life you love doing that's totally unrelated to your work and relationships?

DECIDE

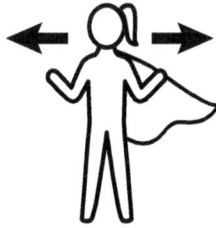

To make time in your day to do activities that bring you joy.

To apologise when it's the right thing to do and feel proud of yourself for doing so.

To not avoid difficult conversations and to learn from them. Practise some of the 8 communication tips listed above.

ACT

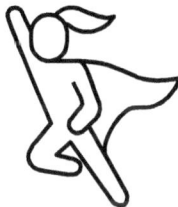

Show appreciation and gratitude for all the positive things in your life. List some things you are grateful for.

....

....

....

....

....

....

....

....

....

....

List some creative things that help you express your true self.

....

....

....

....

....

....

....

....

Make a wish list of fun and exotic things you'd love to do. Instead of a bucket list, maybe make a 'live-life-now' list and explore some new experiences.

Materialising Your Dreams

"

OUR INTENTION CREATES OUR REALITY.

"

Dr Wayne Dyer

Purpose

I heard this quote once: "you can have everything, you just cannot do everything." This has taken me many many years to understand and accept. As I thought my superpower was to do everything. This led to burnout and unhappiness.

The purpose for this chapter is that my journey and experience will help you to be on purpose and not fall into the same traps that I did. To clearly know what you want and to have it.

Check out Alison's personal video to you, the reader, about Superpower 4 in the bonus interactive book. Go to **deanpublishing.com/alisonwheeler** to discover more.

"

YOUR DREAM IS A REALITY THAT IS JUST WAITING FOR YOU TO MATERIALIZE IT!

"

Steve Maraboli

As a child, were you considered a daydreamer with your head in the clouds?

In our youth, we don't always appreciate what a magical, yet fleeting time our childhood is—that special time in our lives when we have the freedom to dream big and believe anything is possible. A time we can dream without fear and imagine without limits.

When we become adults, life becomes more serious, and often we put those dreams on the backburner. We stop dreaming and start conforming. We get told to stop being dreamers, to live in the real world, to get a reality check.

As we become adults, so many of us just robotically live life and do what we think society expects us to do. We do the expected thing rather than follow the dreams in our hearts.

However, I believe that you can design and create the life you want. All it takes is the time to work out what you want and the courage to fail and keep on trying.

For as long as I can remember I have been designing the life I want. There have been times when I lost focus on my vision and every time that happened, I felt like a ship without a rudder — it was directionless. If I lack motivation and direction, then I feel like I'm going around in circles. That circular pattern makes me feel rubbish and I think, because of my own experience with this, I've always had a desire to help others design the life they want and show them the keys that I have used.

CREATE YOUR VISION

I believe the way to design your life is to first have a clear vision. You must create that vision for yourself and not let other people shape it for you.

Having a vision for your life and setting goals to achieve that vision has been associated with:

- Increased feelings of well-being[1]
- Higher levels of energy and vitality[2]

- Greater levels of living with meaning and purpose[3]
- Decreased symptoms of depression.[4]

In short, we generally feel better when we set a vision for our life and go about crafting it into reality.

Having a vision of your future life isn't about useless dreaming, it's about having an intention for your life and staying focused on that intention. In fact, a study[5] revealed that when young people were guided to visualise and experience their future self, they made important connections between their current identity and their future self and therefore worked harder and attained better grades than those young people who didn't have a connection between their current self and future self.

You see, once you have that vision, that's what you choose to focus on and indulge in. That's where your energy goes towards. Now, of course, the journey is not always going to be a straightforward one and there will be challenges along the way, but you won't be directionless. You will be travelling somewhere meaningful. As poetically summed up by Harvard Business School professor and bestselling author Rosabeth Moss Kanter, she said: "A vision is not just a picture of what could be; it is an appeal to our better selves, a call to become something more. To stay ahead, you must have your next idea waiting in the wings."

I love that concept—to have your next idea waiting in the wings. What's waiting in the wings for you? Maybe the difference between those who realise their dreams and those that don't is the seriousness in which they take those 'next ideas' or as I call them my crazy breadcrumb ideas.

Life is filled with plenty of stories of people who have overcome disadvantages to realise their visions and enjoy great success. And of course, there are also plenty of stories about those who didn't make it. Persistence is the key.

I believe we all have a choice about what we're going to focus on and indulge in. If you indulge in a victim story and focus on the unfair things that have happened to you, you will be thrown off your game. You need to go back to the vision you have created for yourself and remember why you want to achieve it. Remember that you're worth achieving it, that you're capable of achieving.

Oprah Winfrey's story is perhaps one of the best known and most amazing. She is an example of someone who drew on her resilience and other deep personal resources and indulged in a new picture, creating an entirely new and positive vision for herself.

Oprah was born into poverty in rural Mississippi to a single teenage mother. She was sexually abused during her childhood and early teens and became pregnant at the age of fourteen. Her son was born prematurely and died in infancy.

Oprah went on to finish high school and through her determination and perseverance, went on to earn a scholarship to college. She began work at a local media network in Nashville and worked her way up the ladder to her status as an international TV star.

Despite all of her obstacles, Oprah stayed steadfast to her dreams and goals and created an astonishing and valuable life for herself. As we all know, she went on to become one of the world's most well-known and influential women of all time.

I've also changed course many times in my life and my process for choosing the best path and materialising my dreams has been tweaked along the way. But that's okay. Life is always changing too.

Like all of us, I didn't exactly know how my life was going to turn out and I went through phases of wanting to be a nurse or a pilot. However, as I grew older, my dreams became less childlike and I knew there was something else I was destined for. I just didn't know what it was.

Even though money was sometimes tight growing up, my parents went above and beyond when it came to the time they invested in their children. They gave me the opportunity to explore everything from athletics to rowing. If my parents didn't have the money to fund an activity, I'd do anything I could to make something happen and realise my dreams. For example, if I wanted to upgrade my bike I would find ways to make money—from selling homemade lemonade and crafts to doing odd jobs.

To cover the costs of rowing, I had a paper round at the age of ten, I worked in a service station and at the local supermarket.

It was a fun game for a while, coming up with all these schemes of making money, until it began to impact my choices about what I was going to do. Growing up, I was always looking for some sort of guidance from my parents, and their response was always, "we just want you to be happy".

As much as I appreciate the fact my parents never put pressure on me, I believe children need something more tangible to aim for when they're growing up because happiness is intangible and sometimes it's hard to discern between instant gratification over long-term happiness.

Dreams also, as much as they're wonderful to have, especially when you're growing up, can seem intangible and often out of reach. So the question is—how do we turn our dreams into a reality?

Recently, I told my husband that I wanted to go for *"a big ass goal in my business"* and make $200,000 profit in a month. This had been my goal for at least five years and although I had come close, I hadn't achieved it yet. My husband didn't think I could do it, but I felt the planets were aligning for me and that this could come together. I said to my husband, *"Look I'm going for this goal and I don't want to hear anything else. You might have a different opinion. That's cool but keep it to yourself for the next thirty days."*

It was okay that my husband didn't believe I could do it because it was my goal and it wasn't his job to believe me. It was important for me to remember that this was a goal that was part of my vision and I didn't need other people to validate it. It was up to me to do this.

I did achieve my goal. And I believe it's because I remained steadfast in not needing validation from others. I didn't need criticism either. I built a shield around me that couldn't be penetrated by others' opinions nor could be disarmed by self-doubt. I stayed focused and refused to take my eyes off the goal I had set for myself.

DREAMS VERSUS VISIONS

I think it's important to understand the difference between dreams and visions. We all have dreams but how many of us actually fulfil them? We tend to idolise people who have actually realised their dreams but what about your dreams? It's important to remember that each person's definition of success is different, as is the path to take them there.

What is the difference between a dream and a vision? We often use the two words interchangeably, but they are actually two different concepts.

Dreams—are inward looking, aspirational and ephemeral. They are something deeply personal and were quite often created when we were young without the experience of life behind us. Dreams are ideas, imaginings and emotions we experience when envisaging what we could potentially have or do.

Visions—are more tangible and outward looking. They tend to be enduring, structured and rooted in daily living, rather than in wishful thinking. A vision is the ability to see something in the future or plan ahead. A vision is often coupled with a plan and goals.

It is however possible for dreams and visions to coexist. There are countless examples where people have turned a dream into a tangible vision and reality.

The key is to structure your dream into something that inspires action and momentum, and this requires intention.

Actor Jim Carey tells a powerful story about never letting go of dreams. When he was fourteen years old his father lost his job and his family hit rough times.

They lived in a caravan on a relative's property and at a young age he took on a factory job to help make ends meet. He quit school at the age of sixteen to focus on comedy full-time and experienced plenty of set-backs and disappointments. Carey moved to Los Angeles shortly afterwards and would park his car on Mulholland Drive every night, taking in all the glamour and visualising the success he had been dreaming of all his childhood.

To make his dream feel more real, on one such night he wrote himself a cheque, made out for $10,000,000, for 'acting services rendered'. He dated it Thanksgiving 1995. Shortly after that Jim Carey was signed up as one of the lead actors in the movie, *Dumber and Dumber*, and was able to cash that cheque.

Success and dream creation come down to how much you believe in yourself. Not just occasionally but every day.

Jim Carrey didn't just dream about his potential life. He showed up to auditions, he practised his craft, he had setbacks and failures. But he kept going!

Failures, disappointments and hearing "no" are all part of realising your vision, but it all depends on how you deal with them and if you're able to learn from them.

Have a clear vision which will give you focus and fulfilment. A vision means you know where you're going no matter how rough the road is ahead of you. That you keep walking the road regardless of the obstacles in your path.

Be clear about your strengths and weaknesses and don't be afraid to enlist the support of others who are able to complement your skills.

INTENTION IS THE KEY

According to Richard Branson, the key to success is intention—"You won't be successful without explicitly knowing what your intentions are every day. The key to success is not only productivity and motivation but intention. Whether you're simply going for a jog or starting a business, intention is the driving force."[6]

Like Richard Branson, I think you really need to know what you want out of life and then create a picture of that. You can keep going back to that intention and hold on to that vision with everything you have, because that's what's going to guide you through. You might make the most micro teeny tiny incremental steps towards that every day, or every other day, and it even may seem like it's painstakingly slow at times, but you are still moving towards it.

Every time you get knocked off course, you need to go back to that vision because that is one of the only things you can control—the vision you hold in your own mind and the steps you take towards it.

It's important to remember that you can't control what anyone else does. You can't control what's happening in the world right now, but you can still create a vision of what you want, and you're able to move towards that every day.

Progress will vary and each day will be different. Some days you take big, significant leaps and other days tiny ones, or no steps at all but as long as you're still moving towards your vision, you're making progress.

> *"THE MAN WHO MOVES A MOUNTAIN BEGINS*
> *BY CARRYING AWAY SMALL STONES."*
> **CONFUCIUS**

STAYING THE COURSE

To stay the course when things get tough, it's important to start every day fresh and not dwell on things that went wrong yesterday. Get your mind ready for the day ahead without focusing on the past. The past is past so you only have today anyway. Get your mind right!

Four ways to stay on track when confronted with an obstacle or delay is to:

1. **Write your intentions down.**

   It may sound simple but writing down your intentions is a sure-fire way to convert them from intentions into actionable goals. For example, you may write—Today I intend to finish two pages of my book. Or, this week I intend to exercise three times per week. Psychology professor, Dr. Gail Matthews discovered that people who wrote down their goals were 42% more likely to achieve their goals than those who didn't write them down.[7] In fact, some highly successful people write down their goals every day! For example, global entrepreneur Grant Cardone writes down his goals TWICE a day.[8]

2. **Use your time wisely and productively.**

   No one has more time than anyone else. Some people have more demands placed on them however (think working mother with three children). When you have lots of demands, it means you need to be ultra- clear about what is worth your time and what isn't. Use the time you have in a way that still moves you forward towards your goals. Planning, organising, delegating and prioritising are all important time management skills.

Research from *Harvard Business Review*, spanning six countries of around 20,000 people clearly showed that working longer hours did not equal higher levels of productivity.[9]

In fact, it showed that both experience and knowing what to focus were the essential master skills. It wasn't adding time to your schedule, it was using the time that you have effectively.

3. **Think ahead.** Thinking ahead is a pattern of a futuristic leader and visionary. Being a thought leader means thinking beyond your immediate situation and planning for what lies ahead. Most great leaders understand that having a vision and a plan are like two wings of a bird, they enable you to fly. Abraham Lincoln was attributed as having said, "If I had four hours to chop down a tree, I'd spend the first two sharpening my axe."

This is planning and vision in one!

4. **Use your imagination.**

Materialising your dream using creative visualisation is a technique in creating what you want in life by using the power of imagination. Using common visualisation techniques can help you convert dreams into future possibilities.

Sports people, for example, use visualisation to calm their nerves, hone their skills and inspire them towards success, excellence and winning.[10] This technique can also be used in business to create goals and aspirations.

VISUALISATION—A TOOL FOR SUCCESS

As an athlete I appreciate how powerful it can be to turn a dream into your reality by actually visualising your victory.

When athletes visualise or imagine a successful competition, they actually stimulate the same brain regions as when they physically perform the same action.

Visualisation in sport, also known as mental imagery, is a way of conditioning for your brain for successful outcomes.

The more you mentally rehearse your performance, the more it becomes ingrained in your mind.

Athletes who use visualisation techniques can reduce performance anxiety and increase mental clarity. Visualisation for athletes is the tool great performers use to help them succeed and stay on top of their game mentally.

Michael Phelps, one of the most decorated Olympians of all time, with twenty-two medals to his name, including eighteen gold, uses guided imagery to prepare for success.

Bob Bowman, Michael Phelps' coach since he was a teenager, has always included mental imagery, or visualisation, as part of his star athlete's mental training.

As part of the training, Bowman instructed Phelps to watch a 'mental video' of his races every day before he went to sleep and when he woke up in the morning.

Phelps would visualise every aspect of his race in great detail: from the starting blocks, to the water entry and turns, to the finish line. Bowman would then instruct Phelps to put in the video tape during training sessions to help motivate him to push harder and develop the habit of success Bowman believes that mental imagery helped Phelps develop the habit of success.

I have used similar techniques throughout my sporting career and found them to be effective.

Recently, I won my professional card in figure bodybuilding which is a top achievement in my sport and means I can compete overseas at the highest level.

However, leading up to the competition, I was feeling disillusioned and looking for answers—what was the next step I needed to take? I knew there was an answer so, to find it, I visualised winning my professional card, with the sash, plate and special crown and found the right people to assist me.

I kept that vision in my head during the competition and ended up winning my special crown which was exciting!

Mental imagery is not just limited to competitive sports. You can also use visualisation in other aspects of your personal and professional life.

Visualise the outcome you want and see the event as how you want it to unfold. If your mental image turns negative, stop the tape and rewind it-restart and then visualise again to see the performance you want to see.

Practice your visualisation or imagery daily.

DESIGN THE LIFE YOU WANT

One of the habits in Stephen Covey's best-selling book, *Seven Habits of Highly Effective People* is to begin with the end in mind. He explains to his readers that "to begin with the end in mind means to start with a clear understanding of your destination. It means to know where you are going so you better understand where you are now and so that the steps you take are always in the right direction."[11]

Having a clear idea of what you want to achieve and being able to prioritise multiple aspirations into a single sustainable main goal is one way to strategically work with your dreams and turn them into reality.

Fixing a goal that is challenging but not impossible and unattainable motivates us to work towards our vision.

SET KEY MILESTONES

When mountain climbers set out, mentally they don't start climbing from the bottom of the mountain. They look at where they want to go and work backwards. They set their eyes on the vision.

It's the same for goal-setting. When you begin with the end in mind and set an action plan, you can begin to work backwards and set interim goals which advance you towards your vision. It doesn't matter if you only do little bit by little bit, step by step, it's about keeping in the game that matters.

> *"REMEMBER TO CELEBRATE MILESTONES AS YOU PREPARE FOR THE ROAD AHEAD."*
> **NELSON MANDELA**

MONITOR PROGRESS

One of the benefits of a structured approach to goal and vision setting is monitoring how each action and effort propels you towards their ultimate goal. It's good to keep a record of your progress, that could be in the form of a journal or specific measurements or data. You can't monitor what you don't measure, so measuring your small wins is important to maintain motivation. As Zig Ziglar said: "I don't care how much power, brilliance or energy you have, if you don't harness it and focus it on a specific target, and hold it there you're never going to accomplish as much as your ability warrants."

ENLIST SUPPORT

Being realistic about what you're able to achieve on your own is also important when it comes to achieving your dreams. Surrounding yourself with and enlisting the support of good people who respect you and share your passion is vital. Having the right people in your corner is essential to your success. No person is an island; so having a supportive network of like-minded people is important to your wellbeing.

Studies have shown that strong social connections in our life, increases our lifespan, strengthens our immune systems and helps us cope with the ups and downs of life better.

KNOW WHEN TO MOVE ON

Goal attainment is linked to current reality so it's important to know when to move on don't be a dreamer who spends all their time dreaming and not actually achieving. Unachievable dreams will suck up your energy and creativity so set realistic and achievable aspirations. There's no point in wanting to be a Rockstar is you've never taken singing lessons or done a gig. Fantasising about your dreams isn't the same as trying to achieve them. True goals require action and passion. I'm a big believer in not giving up on dreams, to not let self-doubt or worry erode the vision of your life, but there is a time to let some dreams go. For example, if you've lost the spark in your heart and no longer feel fulfilled by the dream you've had. Or perhaps you now work in the industry you dreamed of and discover that it wasn't what you imagined. It's okay to tweak your dreams or spark new ones. You don't need to be a hostage to your dreams, you are the dreamer and you get to create them according to your desires.

MY CLIENT'S STORY

Jeanine, a business client I was working with came to me because she was struggling with a rather large monetary milestone she had set for herself—to make $100,000 in a month.

Although she had set the goal, she had actually spooked herself and lost confidence, finding all sorts of reasons why she wouldn't be able to achieve it.

I explained to her that she had placed too much significance on her ultimate goal and that she needed to strip it back, breaking it down into manageable steps.

I encouraged her to visualise those small achievable steps and take one each day towards her goal. When my client was able to visualise her goal in this way, she became more confident about achieving it and was able to properly focus on what she needed to do.

It wasn't that Jeanine couldn't achieve her goal (which she did by the way) but when she looked too far ahead it appeared insurmountable to her. Although having a big vision is great, breaking that big vision down into achievable steps releases the pressure and allows the focus points to be on the next step rather than everything, all at once. I guess this is why the great Desmond Tutu wisely said, "there is only one way to eat an elephant: a bite at a time."

UNLEASHING YOUR FOURTH SUPERPOWER
DESIGNING THE LIFE YOU WANT

REFLECT

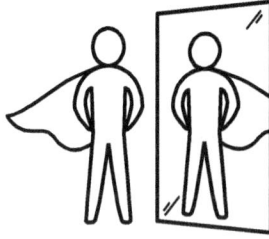

What were your childhood dreams? What are your current dreams?

....

....

....

....

....

....

....

....

....

....

....

....

Think of the life you want. What does it look like and who does it include? Write it in detail.

Write down your ideal day/week. What are you doing? Who is there with you? How do you spend your time?

DECIDE

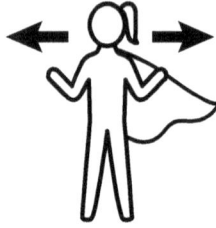

What steps do you need to take to realise your dreams and design the life you want?

Decide to chart your progress whether in the form of a journal or spreadsheet or writing small wins in your calendar. Measure your progress.

ACT

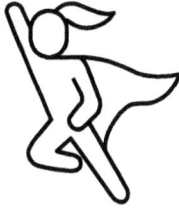

Do at least one solid action within 48 hours that will bring you closer to your goal. It might be to book in for that personal development course you've always wanted to do, or hire a personal trainer and transform your body, or start writing your book. Whatever it is—ACT on it now.

Make a detailed action plan for the next six months that will help you move towards your dreams.

Month 1

....

....

....

....

....

....

....

....

....

....

....

....

....

Month 2

....

....

....

....

....

....

....

....

....

....

....

....

....

Month 3

_____

_____

_____

_____

_____

_____

_____

_____

_____

_____

_____

_____

_____

Month 4

_____

_____

_____

_____

_____

....
....
....
....
....
....
....

Month 5

....
....
....
....
....
....
....
....
....
....

Month 6

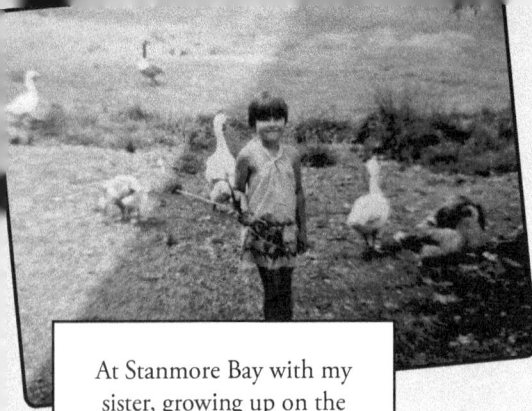

At Stanmore Bay with my sister, growing up on the beach was idyllic.

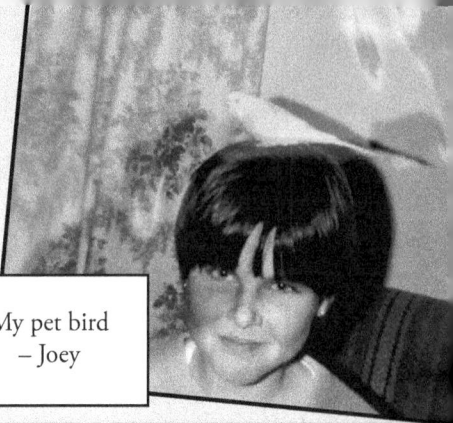

My pet bird – Joey

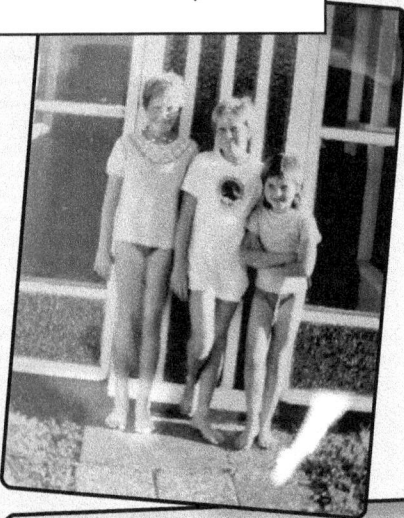

My first day of intermediate school – which is the equivalent of Year 7

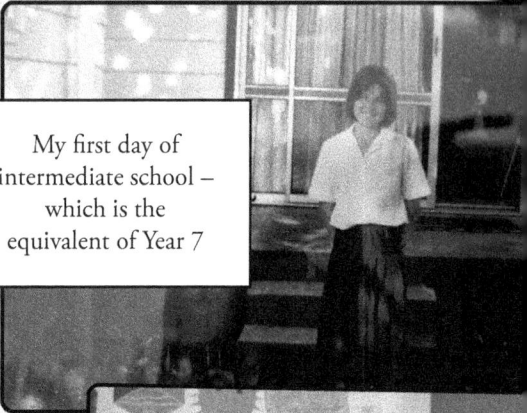

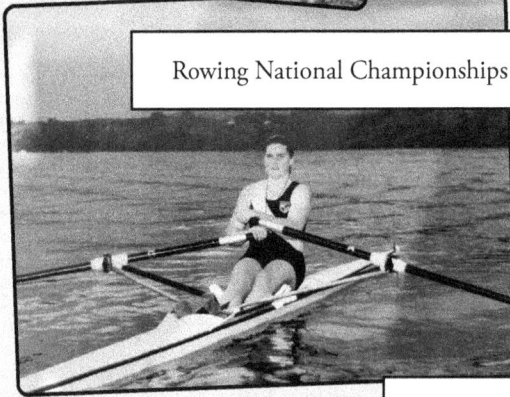

Rowing National Championships

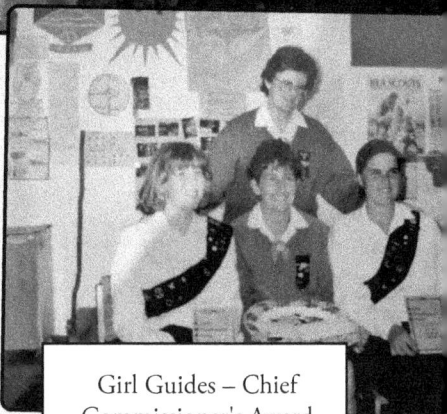

Girl Guides – Chief Commissioner's Award

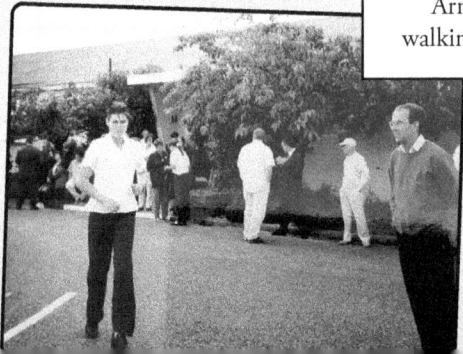

Army training – walking across to Dad

RAYMOND GEORGE NOBLE
(RAY)
20 May 1954 – 8 July 2005

My beautiful Dad

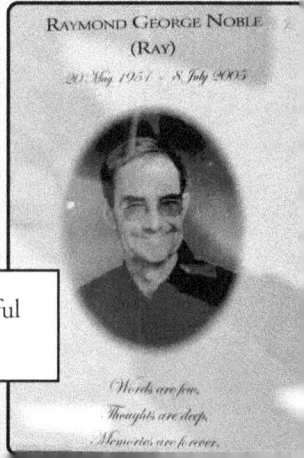

Words are few,
Thoughts are deep,
Memories are forever.

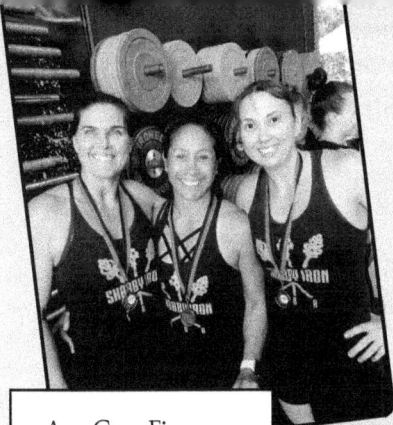

At a CrossFit comp
with my friends

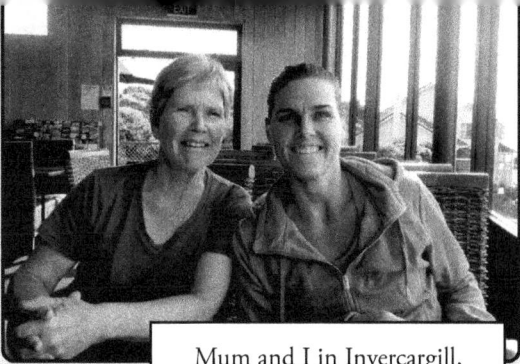

Mum and I in Invercargill,
New Zealand

Me presenting
to a room
of 500+
entrepreneurs

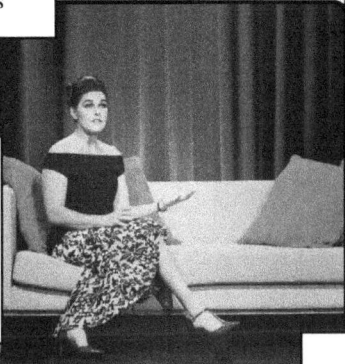

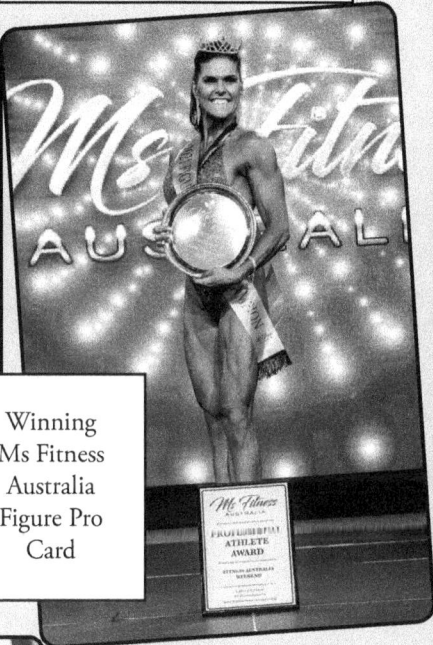

Winning
Ms Fitness
Australia
Figure Pro
Card

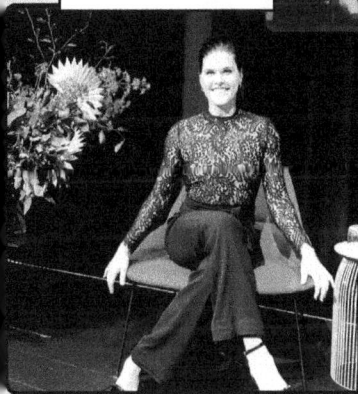

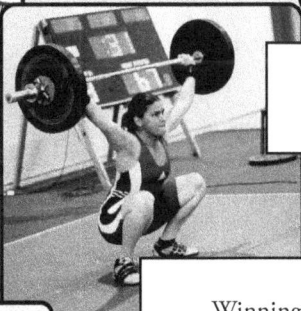

Olympic weightlifting
Queensland championships

Walking on the
beach as a family in
Phuket

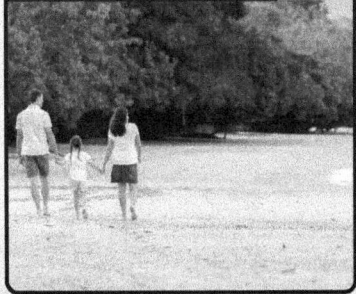

Winning
a 100K
club trophy
business award
($100k profit
in 30 days)

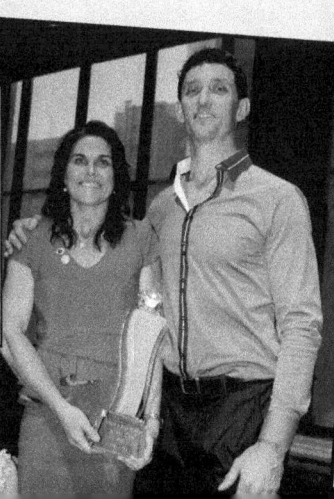

"

DON'T LET YOUR DREAMS JUST BE DREAMS.

"

Jack Johnson

Intuition and Magic

"

INTUITION IS
A SPIRITUAL
FACULTY AND
DOES NOT
EXPLAIN,
BUT SIMPLY
POINTS THE WAY.

"

Florence Scovel Shinn

Purpose

The purpose for this chapter is to
understand that your cup of life is
always full of things: thoughts, actions,
life, you, family, and the list goes on.
You choose what is in your cup of life.
Sometimes your cup is overflowing
and not in a way that serves you.

I hope that through this chapter you can
identify and clean your cup out, keep
what you wish to be in there, and
allow yourself the space to hear the
inner you—the intuitive and magical
part of you, and life.

Check out Alison's personal video to you,
the reader, about Superpower 5 in the
bonus interactive book. Go to
deanpublishing.com/alisonwheeler
to discover more.

"

OWNING OUR
STORY AND
LOVING
OURSELVES
THROUGH THAT
PROCESS IS
THE BRAVEST
THING THAT
WE'LL DO.

"

Brené Brown

The saying goes, "You can't pour from an empty cup." Wise words we're all familiar with, but what do they actually mean?

Essentially, what this is saying is that you can't help others and be productive if you're totally exhausted and your 'cup' is empty—you have nothing left to give.

I must admit, I have tried to pour from an empty cup several times throughout my life and paid the price. Looking back over that time, I can see that my instincts and intuition were trying to tell me something, but I simply wasn't listening.

When things were very difficult for me in high school because of bullying, I poured myself into rowing. At the time, the sporting environment was a place that felt safe for me and I created a lot of success and I created a lot of success. In many ways, it filled my cup: the sense of belonging, the camaraderie, the success. But it also meant very early training sessions, followed by a school, followed by more training school, and pushing my body and mind to the limits.

One particular day, I was in an important rowing race, a final, when I experienced what I can only describe as an out-of-body experience. I was rowing as hard as I could but I simply couldn't push myself any further. It was like I had pushed myself to the point where it seemed I separated my body and mind. Somehow I was outside of my body and seeing myself from the outside. I was wondering why I couldn't push further. It was a surreal experience, and not surprisingly, shortly after that incident, I was diagnosed with glandular fever and spent months off school. Needless to say, my cup was no longer full. I was surprised it was still intact.

Many years later, when I was juggling university with army officer training, I experienced another full-blown empty cup moment. My body and mind end up depleted.

There were some aspects of the army training that I loved, aspects which filled my cup: the team camaraderie and being surrounded by people driven individuals who wanted to excel too.

However, I worked out early on that this was not an environment where individuality was respected and encouraged. In the army it's all about group thinking; you can't stand out. This meant doing better than your fellow recruits was 'beaten out' of you.

Psychologically, it was a vicious circle. The better you did, the more you got hammered and the more pressure they put on you.

When I returned to Otago to continue university, I just couldn't cope with the real world anymore and felt totally out of control. In response, I turned to running which I did really well at but that wasn't enough to make me feel in control.

The next thing I thought I could control was eating and so began my struggle with a serious eating disorder. The illness became so serious I remember contacting my mother and begging her to bring me home before I died.

She flew down immediately, helped me pack my bags and brought me home to heal.

As a result, I had to apply for a medical discharge from the army which was not a straightforward process. So began a cycle of medication, psychologists and psychiatrists as my once strong, athletic body became so emaciated, I was literally just skin and bones.

I was so sick I ended up being medicated but I knew this wasn't solving the underlying internal issue. Even if I followed the advice of my psychologists, I knew I wasn't fixing the real problem and I knew then that I had to find a way out of this terrible illness myself. Medication can work for some, but it just didn't work for me.

My parents were extremely worried about me and wanted to hospitalise me. My father was finding it very hard to cope with seeing his once strong, athletic daughter so weak and debilitated. Interestingly, he turned to running in an effort to deal with his own emotions.

Although my parents did everything they could to support me during this time, including showing me a lot of 'tough love,' they simply didn't understand what I was going through.

How could they? This is such a complex and secretive disease and people around you can't understand how you could be doing such terrible damage to yourself.

This horrendous struggle went on for several years and I was really starting to damage my body, including my teeth, every time I binged.

My eating disorder was also harming people I loved.

It was only when my father said to me one day—*"Look, I literally vomit when I run because this worry is making me sick—"* I knew I had to take back control of the horrible situation I was in. It was tearing us all to pieces.

So, I started to try and find my own way out of it which meant working out the emotional triggers behind this disorder and how to manage them. As I worked through my flawed thought processes, I realised food and eating, for me, had become all about control and that I needed to find a better way to manage life.

Despite my illness, I was still continuing at university and had switched to studying sports science. I then discovered occupational therapy, which I really enjoyed and eventually created a career out of it.

Gradually, I was starting to find my way out of the destructive cycle I was in and reached the stage where I realised, I simply didn't need this in my life anymore.

Of course, my recovery was not as simple as this and whilst I began developing a better relationship with myself, I knew I would have to constantly monitor my choices around food and not use it as a form of control.

I realised I had to use food to nurture and heal my body and be aware of all the triggers that could cause me to fall back into this unhealthy cycle of using food as a form of punishment. I had to really learn how to fill my cup physically, mentally, emotionally and spiritually.

I thank my husband for supporting me in this struggle. Paul understood the disorders and my thinking around food. Like a lot of us, I had grown up being told I had to eat was put in front of me. Paul, on the other hand, respected my choices around food and was willing to travel to the other side of town, if necessary, so I could have the food that nourished me.

KEEPING YOUR CUP FULL

In a world that values productivity and success, looking after ourselves self-care is so often overlooked. We keep pushing ourselves to achieve that we get to the stage where we discover we have nothing left to offer—our cup is empty.

I learnt this the hard way and have had to become very aware of my limits and know when it's time to focus on self-care.

This is particularly true for women today, many of whom are juggling demanding jobs, together with families and still feel they must meet the traditional expectations of what it means to be a 'good wife and mother.'

As women, we are also brought up to believe that it's our role to nurture and look after others and that putting ourselves first is selfish.

So how do you find that balance between realising your goals but also ensuring your cup remains full?

The lessons I learnt when I was dealing with my own serious health challenges was that it is so important to listen to what your body is trying to tell you and not ignore the warning signs, before it's too late.

You cannot realise your goals and achieve success when you are physically and mentally empty.

THE MYTH OF SELFISHNESS

I believe in our society, there's a misconception about what selfishness actually means.

We tend to define a selfish person as someone who lacks consideration for other people and puts themselves first—only concerned about their own profit or pleasure.

But I sometimes wonder, is putting yourself first selfish or selfless?

Being selfless means you are more concerned with the needs and wishes of others than your own. However, I think, to a certain degree, if you're not putting yourself first, you are actually being selfish.

The reason I say that is because when you are being selfless, your cup ends up empty and has nothing left to offer.

Girls, in particular, are taught from an early age that everyone else's needs come first. This is a really bad lesson to teach them. If girls follow this lesson into their adult life, inevitably they will feel they have to keep giving and giving, ending up an empty shell.

I think women can so easily fall into the trap of becoming a martyr, especially when they become mothers. You know society has certain expectations of you and that's a role you're expected to pay and that if you don't do it properly in other people's eyes, or refuse to take on certain parts of this role, you may be judged and shamed.

On the other hand, I also think that for many women there is also an issue of control when it comes to 'selfishness'. This is because, at some level, they think they must do everything on their own because no one else will do it to their standard.

Often this happens without us realising so it's so important to be honest about these underlying thoughts that influence your behaviour. It's also important to be willing to let go of certain things and allow others to help you.

UNDERSTANDING EGO

To a certain extent this willingness to let go and surrender some control is about understanding our egos.

I think martyrdom is a role women readily take on, especially once they become mothers.

Is this about being selfless or more about our egos?

I believe we have a mixed-up idea of what ego is. We think it means being egotistical—those people who puff out their chests and think they're awesome. That may be one side of what ego means but, once again there is a flip side.

This is the pressure you put on yourself to be all things to all people. This habit feeds your ego in a negative sense, until your cup runs dry.

This is a side of our egos that's not very well explored, nor understood, but it's still about being egotistical.

As women, at some point in time, you have to be willing to challenge your ego and break this stereotype. Challenge all the social conditioning you have been exposed to growing up and stop feeding that side of your ego that needs control. This means choosing a different path which is often not easy.

Because I believe being selfless means you are concerned more with the needs and wishes of others than with your own. I think it to a degree, if you're not putting yourself first, that is being selfish, because you end up with nothing to give.

In some ways, that is also about control because on some level you think that you've got to do it on your own, which means that you think other people can't do it. You have to kind of face those underlying thoughts that you have going on and be willing to let go.

There's so much conditioning and social expectations around what it means to be a 'good mother' but at some point, you have to be willing to break that stereotype and stop feeding that ego side that has bought into the martyr story. You need to disagree with that story which is not an easy thing to do.

Being a so-called good mother isn't about denying your needs and serving others—that's close to the definition of a slave. Award-winning author and social justice activist L.R. Knost. summed it up beautifully when she said, " Taking care of myself doesn't mean 'Me First', it means 'Me Too.'"

SELF-DISCIPLINE VERSUS SELF-PUNISHMENT

Growing up, my parents and other people kept asking me—*"Why are you so driven?"* It was almost as if this was something wrong, something I had to apologise for.

Although I would exercise because it's something I love to do, however, when I look back to those times when I reached burnout, I realised that I was using it as a form of punishment because I wasn't getting the results I wanted and becoming frustrated.

This meant I wasn't using my training to nurture and fulfil myself, but rather as a way to beat myself up.

The challenge for me was to try and find a balance between my natural drive and knowing when to slow down to avoid burning out. This was not easy for me as, growing up, I had been criticised for being so driven and that this was something frowned upon.

Then I discovered a book by American entrepreneur and author, Brian Tracy, *No Excuses! The Power of Self Discipline*1, and it really was an eye-opener to me because it validated my whole approach to life.

After reading this book, I finally realised being me was totally okay and that there were other successful people in the world following the way I do things. I realised the reason I was in the cycle of pushing myself to exhaustion was because I kept trying to fight something that came so naturally to me. It wasn't until I stopped resisting and accepted that having so much drive and determination was actually a good thing and I didn't have to feel flawed. By accepting this, I was able to let go of all the shitty, self-sabotaging behaviour I had indulged in over the years and stop resisting. I could indulge in being me. Once I stopped resisting and gave up the fight, I felt more in flow.

According to Brian Tracy, the reason many of us don't achieve our goals is because we lack self-discipline.

Tracey argues even an average person can achieve miracles with self-discipline and that without it, even the luckiest and most talented person won't rise above mediocrity.

In his book Tracy urges his readers to start acting today to build their own happiness, by applying the many teachings he has fine-tuned over the years.

For a rewarding life you need to constantly improve yourself and plan your actions with this seven-step method.

7 STEPS TO IMPROVE YOUR LIFE IMMEDIATELY

1. Define your goal exactly and be specific. For example, if you want to save money, work out how much.
2. Write down your specific goals.
3. Set a realistic deadline. If a goal is complicated to achieve or requires a lot of time, break it up into sub-tasks, setting a deadline for each.

4. Think of the obstacles you may face in the process and the resources you think you may need to succeed, including skills and what steps you need to take to acquire them.
5. Organise your list sequentially, prioritising the most beneficial task that must be completed first.
6. Start today with your first step.
7. Do something every day, even small, to get a little closer to your goal.

ALL ABOUT INTENTION

Arguably, being so driven and focused on success may become a form of self-punishment, for some of us, especially if you push yourself to the point of exhaustion and burnout.

However, I think this depends on the vision you have of your success and whether you are enjoying what you're doing.

I don't see my drive and hard work as self-punishment, because it fits my vision and I love what I'm doing. I don't always enjoy every aspect of it because everything you do has parts you won't like. However, for me it's about nurturing myself and evolving my potential.

On the other hand, I have the tendency to be anxious and I have to monitor when things trigger me because that's when my self-discipline and drive can easily flip into an anxiety response, and self-punishment. That's something I need to be very mindful of.

Whilst I may be really enjoying what I'm doing, sometimes I realise I might be starting to push myself a bit too hard, possibly punishing myself, rather than enjoying what I'm doing. I observe myself carefully to ensure I stay in the realm of passion and pleasure and not in the realm of self-punishment.

It all comes back to the intention behind your actions because anything could become self-punishment. The question to ask yourself is, *Am I doing this to reprimand myself, or to move towards my goal?* I think you fall over faster if you're doing it from a position of self-punishment.

Admittedly, there can be a fine line between the two, and you need to be aware of this, especially if you're a driven individual. Once again, this comes back to listening to and respecting your intuition.

FINDING YOUR OKAY SPACE

I think we all intuitively know where that 'okay space' is inside us and should be aware when we're doing something to punish ourselves.

Similarly, with your body and physical health. You can push your body to test its limits and see what it's capable of and be rewarded with the satisfaction of achieving your best. But if you possibly push it that little bit too hard, you can injure yourself and that could become a form of self-punishment.

Self-punishment can encompass a whole range of behaviours, including:
- negative self-talk
- scolding yourself when we've made a mistake
- engaging in destructive activities, such as drug taking
- restrictive eating or overeating
- feeling guilty over every little thing you failed to do
- denying yourself gratification because you think you don't deserve it
- over-exercising or not exercising at all
- neglecting yourself and your needs
- sabotaging your happiness or potential opportunities.

People most likely to engage in self-punishment are those who are highly sensitive to the perceptions of others and worry about their reputation. Do you fall into this category?

Interestingly, those who feel it's important to take responsibility for their actions often end up engaging in mental self-punishment, by beating themselves about something they did or didn't do.

It's important to know when self-punishment becomes self-sabotage, which is not beneficial.

YOUR INTUITION FOR FILLING YOUR CUP

Although I have discussed the importance of our intuition in previous chapters, I think it's also important to re-emphasise it here. As a culture we tend to put a great deal of emphasis on rationality and what we should be focused on when making important decisions in our lives.

But what about that inner voice inside all of us—that gut feeling from within that speaks to us beneath those layers of logic; our instincts and intuitions. When dealing with self-care, quite often our inner voice has been guiding and nudging us already, but we haven't been listening, or refusing to listen.

Have you heard inner whispers telling you to slow down, or take time out for yourself? Or perhaps your intuition has been nudging you to work part-time or change the pace of your frantic life?

We need both instinct *and* reason to make the best possible decisions for ourselves, our business and our families.

Psychologists describe *instinct* as our innate inclination toward a particular behaviour, as opposed to a learned response.[2]

A gut feeling or a hunch is a certain type of feeling or sensation we experience without the full knowledge of why we feel that way. Usually, there is an unconscious or underlying reason for it that we aren't fully aware of.

Intuition is a process that gives us the ability to know something directly without analytic reasoning—bridging that gap between the conscious and the non-conscious parts of our mind and bridging the gap between instinct and reason.

Unfortunately, many of us are uncomfortable with the idea of basing important decisions on our instincts and embarrassed to say our decision was based on a hunch. This means we tend to ignore the cryptic messages our instincts send to us and diminish the capacity to leverage the power of our own instincts when we need them most.

Including intuition in your everyday life is important. You don't need to dismiss your logic or practicality, but make room for your intuition too.

So, how do we integrate intuition into our decision-making process? Psychologists suggest dialoguing it.

The unconscious mind searches through the past, present and future and connects with hunches in a non-linear way.

The conscious mind is logical and rational and demands our attention. The unconscious process is cryptic and defies conventional laws of time and space.

Listen to your instincts without worrying about the logical reasons why.

DIALOGUING YOUR INNER VOICE

1. Keep a journal writing your thoughts and feelings down on paper. This helps the unconscious mind open up.
2. Turn off your inner critic and don't rationalise away the unconscious thoughts. Allow the inner dialogue to happen without fear of ridicule.
3. Find a peaceful place where you can allow emotions to flow freely.

EMILY—AVOIDING EXHAUSTION

One of my clients Emily, a successful businesswoman and mother, had so much going on in her life, to the point she was managing everyone else and doing what she thought she had to do to succeed. This meant she was starting to neglect her basic needs, including sacrificing sleep to the point of exhaustion. As a result, she was losing the joy in life and needed some help getting back on track.

Working with Emily, we first looked at making sure she was meeting her basic needs—was she eating and drinking enough. These may seem obvious but are often the things people overlook when they're stressed and overworked. I encouraged Emily to move out of the pattern of self-punishment she was in and start nourishing herself more. We made a plan for that first. In many ways, this plan was to detour where she was heading (into burnout) and re-route a new pathway to health and self-care.

Even the Dalai Lama gave advice on this subject. Given the epidemic of people suffering from exhaustion and burnout, he said:

"In dealing with those who are undergoing great suffering, if you feel "burnout" setting in, if you feel demoralized and exhausted, it is best, for the sake of everyone, to withdraw and restore yourself. The point is to have a long-term perspective."

Emily needed to play the long-game and stop neglecting herself. She understood that she needed to concentrate on her fundamental wellbeing first in order to have long-term success.

So Emily started caring for herself physically, she started to move her bedtime forward instead of working until she face-planted in her laptop at night from exhaustion. She ate more nourishing foods and carved some time out of her busy schedule for just her. Then she was able to focus on other priorities, such as building her business and reaching greater financial heights.

She had stopped doing things out of obligation and was now listening to what was actually required. After addressing her basic self-care needs, Emily ended up having a hugely successful month in her business.

UNLEASHING YOUR
FIFTH SUPERPOWER
ENSURING YOUR CUP REMAINS FULL

So often we kid ourselves into thinking we can and must do it all, driving ourselves to exhaustion. To be successful and enjoy a fulfilling life, it's important to ensure your 'cup' is always full.

I encourage you to take some time out of your busy schedule and consider the following:

REFLECT

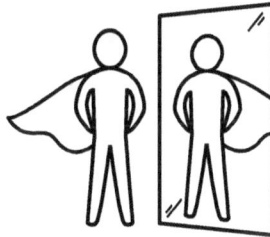

How full is your cup? What's filling it up? What is emptying your cup?. Write down your response.

....

....

....

....

....

....

....

....

....

....

....

....

....

....

....

....

....

....

FILL UP YOUR BUCKET

Is your body trying to get your attention? Are you constantly tired and lacking in energy or full of aches and pains? Write down what your body is trying to tell you. What's the message?

....

....

....

....

....

....

....

....

....

....

DECIDE

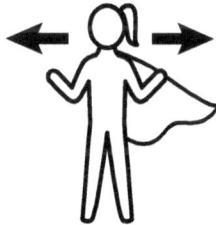

To listen to your body and not ignore physical signs of stress and fatigue.

Do not wait until your 'cup' is completely empty before doing something.

Fill up your cup with nourishing things.

ACT

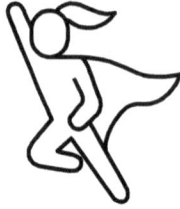

Be prepared to let go of some control. Write down all the ways you can ease the burden and let go of some control.

_____

_____

_____

_____

_____

_____

_____

_____

_____

_____

_____

_____

_____

_____

Let the people around know you're struggling. Ask for help. Write down a list of people, services or places that could provide assistance to you.

....

....

....

....

....

....

....

....

....

....

Prioritise tasks and be willing to delegate to others. Write down all the things you can delegate and to whom.

....

....

....

....

....

....

....

....

....

....

....

....

....

....

....

....

....

....

Name two ways you will fill your cup this week.

1. ....

....

2. ....

....

The Sword of Success

"

LIFE IS
MESSY.
LOVE IT
ANYWAY.

"

Unknown

Purpose

The purpose for this chapter is to understand that life is a messy thing. We can structure and do what we can to help us navigate—this gives us the map. But we are still operating off a compass. That will mean we get off track, we make mistakes and at times cannot see things coming together.

Hold onto your vision my beautiful friend and keep trusting yourself in taking the next step. The story is not over until the very end.

Check out Alison's personal video to you, the reader, about Superpower 6 in the bonus interactive book. Go to **deanpublishing.com/alisonwheeler** to discover more.

"

IT ALWAYS SEEMS IMPOSSIBLE UNTIL IT'S DONE.

"

Nelson Mandela

No matter how much we try to plan and manage it, life can be unpredictable and messy.

In fact, I think people need to understand that success is the messiest thing you're ever going to see.

The greater our ambition, the more complicated and messy life can be, but as I've learnt over the years, you need to embrace the chaos because it's all part of achieving success and it's worth it in the end.

Science has a term for this phenomenon, it's called 'entropy'. A simple scientific definition for *entropy* is—to determine the amount of disorder (chaos) in a closed system.

Some describe this as one of the great forces of our universe—so fundamental it governs all our lives and permeates every endeavour we pursue.

A simple example is when you take a set of puzzle pieces and tip them out of the box. The odds of them falling in correct order to make a completed puzzle is pretty much impossible.

However, science has also taught us that on the other side of this messiness and chaos, there's very often order and beauty.

I believe we can apply these scientific theories to our own lives and learn from them.

Because the universe consists of both order and chaos, you have to continually revisit and work towards recreating your version of success.

One of the most important lessons I've learnt throughout my own journey is that success doesn't happen in a straight line.

In fact, achieving success often involves a convoluted and unpredictable process, with setbacks and disappointments along the way.

Despite this, we tend to have certain expectations about how success should look and become carried away by all the glamorous trappings we associate with being successful.

I think we need to cut through the illusions and fantasy of how success is often portrayed in movies and on social media and accept that it means different things to different people.

I believe it's very important to know what your version of success is— whether it's big or small, it doesn't really matter. It's whatever success means to you because this is your unique vision—no-one else has the blueprint.

I discovered my version of success and how messy the process can be when I went into business with my husband in 2009.

It was not something I planned, but rather was an opportunity that came along at a time in my life when I was looking for a new challenge and perhaps a new vision.

As the saying goes, hindsight is a wonderful thing, and I wish I realised then what I do now about the process of achieving success.

In business, as in sport, you're constantly confronted with pressure to take that next step and improve your performance. Along the way there are disappointments; you get hurt and need time to recover; your competitors may want you to see you fail; one day you're on top and the next day you're considering quitting. It's a messy process! As actor Robert Downey Jr said, "Life is just so painful and messy and hard and worth it and all that stuff." And given his colourful life of ups and downs, I guess he would know.

THE MESSY MIDDLE

Think about the last time you cleaned up your house or carried out a renovation. Your home is going to be chaotic and dirty before it becomes clean and ordered.

This is the same in business, especially when you decide to create a new vision. This is because you have to disturb the existing picture and create a new version of your vision.

There's always going to be a messy period where you're transforming that vision into something new. It's almost unavoidable.

If you look at the messy middle as part of the process, it enables you to be more patient and accept there's going to be a tough messy period you'll have to deal with. This period may be brief or may last a long time but remember to always focus on the beauty and order so you can enjoy the process and make your way to the finish line.

Regardless of how long it lasts and how difficult a process it is, you know that order will be restored when you eventually get to the other side.

When I look back on my own life and all the different roads I have travelled to arrive where I am today, I can appreciate the convoluted path I have taken and what each step has taught me.

From athletics and netball, to rowing and bodybuilding, my sporting career progressed in anything but a straight line.

Similarly, with my career—from studying at university, enrolling in army officer training, followed by a diploma in fitness, occupational health and later reinventing myself as a life coach—mine was clearly not a well-planned career path!

I have also had to deal with plenty of personal and painful setbacks throughout my life, challenging my resolve to achieve the goals I've set myself along the way.

In the sport of bodybuilding, no one sees what actually goes on behind the scenes. They just see the glory and the accolades—the fit bodies, the bikinis, the shiny, glamourous trappings of success.

They don't see all the work that goes in beforehand and the fact there are so many unknowns because you've got no idea how your body is going to respond to the training and how you're going to take that next step, and then the next. There is no defined path and you literally can't see the wood for the trees which can be so frustrating and messy!

It's the same when I'm coaching my clients. Regardless of the challenge they face, I always encourage them to work out what the next step in the process is and what they can do to get closer to it. I assure them that the answers will unfold as they step forward, towards their goal and their vision. Part of life involves a leap of faith and stepping towards our dreams when we don't hold all the answers.

Perhaps some would consider the path my life has taken as being convoluted and chaotic and that I made things unnecessarily hard for myself along the way, but I don't see it that way.

Rather, I would describe it rather as a journey of self-discovery that despite the highs and lows, brought me to where I am now. This is a life which fits my vision and it's where I want to be.

I think it's important to teach and prepare our children for the 'messiness', at least as far as career paths are concerned. According to futurists, by the time my Gen Z daughter finishes her education and joins the workforce, she is statistically likely to have eighteen jobs, spanning six careers and live in fifteen residences![1] My job is to help prepare her for the uncertain and unpredictable world.

FAIL IN ORDER TO SUCCEED

Let's be honest. We all want to be liked and admired and enjoy being around successful people.

However, what people forget is that success takes time and effort and once people have become successful, they may want to leave the hard times behind them.

Successful people may not always tell you about the blunders they've made along the way, about the dark and difficult times that were anything but glamorous. Yet these experiences are just as much a part of their success as the awards and accolades.

The difference between long-term success and failure is how we react to setbacks, disappointments and to the messiness and continue forward anyway.

I think we avoid using the word failure because it's the stark opposite to success and it tends to be associated with shame, so we protect ourselves from it.

In work situations people are often so afraid of being blamed for failures meaning they go unreported and important lessons are lost. Taking responsibility is a big part of this.

No-one wants to experience failure, or be described as a 'failure', yet failure can be the very catalyst for success. This is because it's not always about reaching the destination that defines the person, but the journey you take to get there.

It's all about having the courage to try things that are new or different or perhaps even fly in the face of conventional wisdom but the worst thing that can happen is that you make a mistake which is how you learn and grow.

FAMOUS FAILURES

Some of the most famous successful people in history, from scientists and performers, to sporting icons, have not taken a straight path to success and, in fact, experienced some quite spectacular failures.

As a child, Thomas Edison was thought to be unintelligent. He was told that he would never be a success by many of his teachers because his mind would often wander in class. When asked about the thousand failures he had when trying to create the light bulb, he famously replied, "I have not failed. I have just found ten thousand ways that won't work."

Albert Einstein also did not achieve success and fame easily. He had speech difficulties as a child and was once considered to be mentally handicapped. As a teen he rebelled against the traditional teaching style of rote learning and failed many of his subjects. He famously said, "anyone who never made a mistake has never tried anything new."

Elvis Presley, one of the most successful recording artists in history, failed his music class and, at school, was somewhat of a social misfit. When he tried to join a vocal quartet, he was told he couldn't sing.

Michael Jordan, arguably the greatest basketball player of all time ever, was once cut from his high school team but he kept working at his skills and improving.

As Jordan put it, "I have missed more than nine thousand shots in my career. I have lost almost three hundred games. On twenty-six occasions I have been entrusted to take the game's winning shot and I missed. I have failed over and over again in my life. And that is why I succeed."

Jerry Seinfeld is another inspiring example of someone who embraced his failures and learnt from them. The first time he did a stand-up act at a comedy club he lasted only three minutes and was booed off the stage. Despite this humiliating experience he continued doing what he loved doing—stand-up acts all over New York, eventually becoming one of the greatest American comedians of all time. When asked about his achievements, his simple advice was to "keep your head up in failure, and your head down in success."

PREPARE TO GET MESSY

Whether it's your journey to physical, financial, or even spiritual health, we often think there should be a straight obvious line towards improvement. However, life rarely works that way.

You may plan to achieve something, but the reality is, we're all human and life can be unpredictable, often throwing unexpected obstacles at us.

To change your vision and ideally achieve the success you want, it's almost like you have to pull something apart before you can rebuild it and achieve perfection.

With that process comes an uncomfortableness of the unknown, because you're pulling something apart and putting it all back together—not quite sure where all the pieces go. You also don't know what the outcome is going to look like so there is that uncertainty.

When you form a new relationship, you're both trying to work each other out, as well as the baggage you've both brought to the relationship, and that can be messy!

Bringing home a new baby can also be a wonderfully chaotic time in your life. When my daughter was born, I found transitioning to motherhood very challenging because no one warns you how suddenly it happens and that there's no transitionary period. One minute you're pregnant and the next thing you're a mother!

I'd always been so driven with my career and sport and to have a tiny baby completely dependent on me was quite challenging. At the time, I remember thinking, *who the hell am I now?*

It was a real journey to find myself again and to reinvent myself in my new role as a mother. However, as I adjusted to my new 'normal', amongst the 'messiness' I also found a lot of joy.

As I mentioned with bodybuilding, the competitions may look as though it's all about glamour and amazing bodies, but no one sees what happens behind the scenes and how much work goes into preparing for a competition. Training requires a huge amount of self-discipline and sacrifice. There's also no perfect path for success and it's so easy to go off course.

So how do you see through the fog of chaos and messiness and find a path out?

I believe you need to look for the very next step you can do and then the answers will reveal themselves. It's like the wise words of famed Spanish poet Antonio Machado, "Wanderer, there is no way, the way is made by walking…"

Yes, you need to walk the road to see the next corner. The journey unfolds as you walk.

Now, you may find that you have a vague idea of what you want your final destination of success to look like. You might then start the process of moving puzzle pieces around and discover the combination is not quite right. So, you've got to go back and modify and learn as you grow.

To a certain extent messiness may feel like you have no control of your life and that's a comfortable feeling.

I'm not sure if I'm totally comfortable with success being a messy process but I have to just accept it is an important part of the process.

I've also learnt along the way that, with mess, comes experience. The more messes we have to fix, the more experience we gain.

Once I accepted that messiness was actually an integral part of achieving success and stopped resisting it, I was able to focus on the next thing I could do to take me towards my vision and goals.

I just needed to have the patience to work through the mess, staying committed to my vision and having the courage to take the next step that came to me—right, wrong or otherwise, and to always be willing to find more knowledge.

Once I did that, I knew I would get a little bit more of the picture and work out whether I needed to do a bit of a correction.

I think we need to adjust our perception of success being a straight path to our dreams, and realise that in reality it's more of a windy and bent road of surprises, setbacks and detours. But, yes, it's all worth the adventure in the long-run.

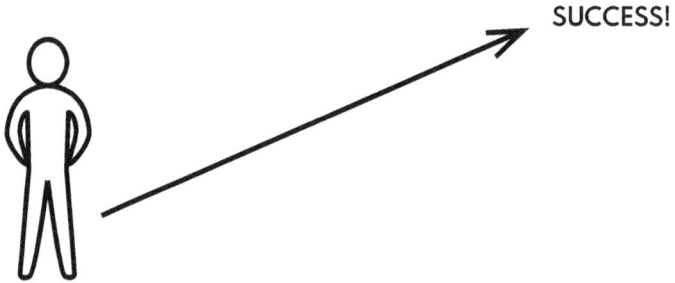

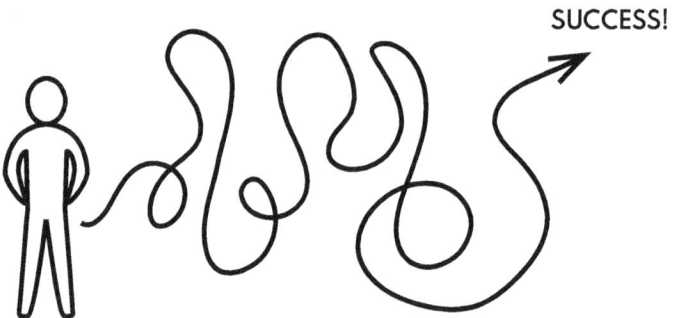

UNLEASHING YOUR SIXTH SUPERPOWER
CHALLENGING YOUR DEFINITION OF SUCCESS AND EMBRACING FAILURE

REFLECT

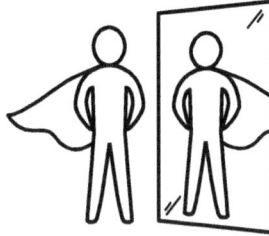

Think about the times you have made mistakes and failed at something. How did it feel and how did you react to the failure? What was the learning?

....

....

....

....

....

....

....

....

....

....

What does success mean to you? Define it clearly.

....

....

....

....

....

....

....

....

....

....

....

....

....

....

Who are three people you really admire?

1. ....

2. ....

3. ....

Why do you admire them?

DECIDE

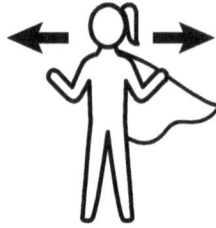

To let failure happen.

To embrace your failures and the messiness of success.

To not allow mistakes and failures derail you from following your vision.

To not worry what other people think of you.

ACT

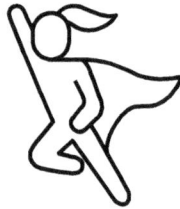

Make note of each time you make a mistake or fail at something.

Write down the lesson(s) you have learnt from this experience.

Make a point of connecting with a person you admire and ask them to tell you about the mistakes they've made along the way and what they've learnt from them.

Make a note of each time to stay committed to your path despite obstacles, how do you embrace the messy road to success along the way?

SUPERPOWER #7

Mind Control

"

YOU EITHER CONTROL YOUR MIND OR IT CONTROLS YOU.

"

Napoleon Hill

Purpose

We all have negative self-talk and demons in our mind. You can leash the demons and therefore unleash a new part of you. In this chapter, we will go on a journey and discover some fundamental and basic truths that will allow you to take control of your mind and your life.

Let's do this!

Check out Alison's personal video to you, the reader, about Superpower 7 in the bonus interactive book. Go to **deanpublishing.com/alisonwheeler** to discover more.

"

IF YOU STOP LISTENING WITH YOUR HEART, THE UNIVERSE WILL STOP GIVING YOU THE MESSAGE.

"

Paulo Coelho, The Alchemist

DREAMS VERSUS DEMONS

We all have one inside us. That persistent, negative inner critic that often won't let up and leave you in peace—*You're not good enough. You're going to fail. You don't deserve to be here.* Does this sound familiar?

But it's important to understand this is a model of reality you've developed in your own head, as a form of punishment and to hold yourself back and keep you safe.

Perhaps there has been someone in your past who has been critical of you and you've now taken that criticism on? That is the demon talking inside your head.

For example, I used to listen to the bullies at school who made me feel less because I didn't easily fit into one of their cliques. I listened to my critics who told me I was "too driven and harsh" in the way I acted and that there was something wrong with me. People would often make comments about my personality, saying things like, "you're harsh" or "you have no feelings" or "why do you have to be so driven?" or "you're fat and ugly"—even though I grew up like that it didn't make the impact of those comments any less harmful.

Battling your inner critic is a major problem for many of us. We all have our demons, and no one is alone when it comes to fighting them.

It doesn't matter how successful you are, or what you have achieved in life. Anyone can fall prey to their inner critic. How well you're able to handle and control these negative messages will determine the outcome for you.

Remember, you have a choice about the type of thoughts you indulge in. You can choose to listen to your demons, let them take over, or you can focus on your goals and dreams. It's entirely up to you because you have the power to choose.

In making that choice, remember, one will feed you, move you forward and make you powerful. The other will suck your life energy and leave you powerless.

It's similar to the famous Cherokee parable where the grandfather is telling his grandson a story and says, "In life, there are two wolves inside of us which are always at battle. One is a good wolf which represents things like kindness, courage, and love. The other is a bad wolf which represents things like greed, hatred, and fear."

The grandson looks at his grandfather with wide-eyed curiosity and says, "Grandfather, which one wins?"

"The one you feed," his grandfather replies.

This is true in today's world too. If you feed the demons of your mind, they will get stronger and stronger. If you starve them of your time, energy and attention—they get weaker and cannot control you.

I'm not suggesting this is an easy choice to make. Sometimes it can be very difficult to take control of those voices in your head, especially when your inner critic insists on dominating the conversation.

When this happens, you literally have to put a timeframe on it, set a timer if you need to and tell yourself, *I'm going to indulge in this shitty thinking for five minutes and then that's enough. I now need to move on to this next thing.* Even if it's a simple distraction, like getting outside for a walk. Whatever you can think of doing to move out of this negative mindset, as long as it's healthy and not destructive.

I encourage my clients to be aware of these negative stories circulating in their heads and understand where they are coming from. I then encourage them to change the story and take action by stopping the war in their mind.

Knowing that you can and will cycle out of this negative mindset and acknowledging no thought is permanent, means you have taken control of the battle and won.

MEETING YOUR BASIC NEEDS

It's important to remember that you can't be in control of your demons if you haven't actually met your basic needs. Your basic needs are things like good nutrition, water, sleep, sunshine, fresh air and connection.

If you start to feel the demons beginning to gang up on you, ask yourself: *have I had enough sleep lately, am I actually hungry, am I eating properly, do I need to get some fresh air?*

They may seem obvious yet so often we overlook and neglect them and end up feeling depleted. This is when we're more likely to give in to our demons. When our basic needs are met, it's much easier to handle our more complex emotional needs.

Do an audit on yourself and check whether you have been neglecting your basic needs. Consider the pressure or stress you've been under and whether this has impacted your sleep, exercise regime or nutrition. Have you been living off fast microwave meals and coffee to keep pace with life? Have you been putting everyone else before yourself and now feel tired and depleted?

Keeping a strong mindset is a whole-body job. What we put into our bodies affect our minds and what we put into our minds affect our bodies. Sleep deprivation is well known to reduce our motivation levels, memory, concentration and cognitive functions.[1] It is also strongly linked with depression, anxiety and other mental health issues.[2]

So looking after your basic needs is essential in building a strong mindset. Too many people try to succeed in life and end up burning themselves out through overwork, overwhelm and exhaustion. I should know because I did this too. But it's a short road. It's like sprinting at your fastest pace in a marathon—eventually you will hit the wall and not make the distance.

Looking after your basic needs is the only way to cross the finish line in this marathon we call life and still be filled with energy, optimism and good health.

So I suggest to all my clients to not overlook the simple things. Take a good hard look at your lifestyle and see if it serves your needs. Do an audit on your life to see if you can perform at optimal levels without burning out or creating a fertile place for demons to breed.

THE 'BASIC NEEDS' AUDIT
- Are you getting adequate sleep?
- Are you nourishing yourself with good nutrition?
- Are your stress levels low to moderate?
- Do you exercise regularly?
- Do you get enough fresh air, sunshine and water?
- Do you have time for yourself to do things you enjoy?

If you answered no to any of these questions, then take control and make an immediate change. A small step in the right direction will pay dividends in the long run.

MEETING THE INNER CRITIC HEAD-ON

One of my clients Kate was a corporate executive, working in a 'man's' world which she found to be an incredibly challenging and tough environment to be in and where she felt her contribution was invalidated. This left her full of self-doubt and uncertainty. She questioned whether she belonged in this tough corporate environment and whether she could compete.

Through my coaching, I helped Kate acknowledge and understand her inner critic. I reminded her that she did not have to agree with her inner critic and that there were techniques she could use to counteract the negative messages it was continually giving her.

I encouraged Kate to write down the story her inner critic was telling her and read it out loud. By doing this she realised how ridiculous and false it really was.

I then told her to rip this old story and write a new story in its place that was more accurate. Kate told me she went through this process and wrote a new story that she revisited every day. Although at the beginning, the old inner critic kept trying to derail her new story, she kept revisiting her new story until she got to the stage where she felt a lot more at ease with it. Over time, Kate became comfortable to express herself in her work environment and she discovered that her ideas were in fact valued amongst her peers and yet she now didn't need others to validate her.

Kate realised that it wasn't her colleagues criticising her, it was herself. She was her own worst enemy. She was the one demanding more of herself and deeming herself incapable. Once she conquered the demons in her own mind, she conquered the root cause of the problem.

BANISHING THE DEMONS

It also helps to verbalise this battle between your demons and dreams or express it in another physical way.

Punch a pillow for five minutes, saying out loud all the rubbish that's in your head. Write it all down on a piece of paper, rip it up and burn it. Anything to get it out of your reality. The more you can put the demons inside your head into a solid form, such as down on paper, the more likely you are to silence them, banishing them from your reality.

Don't be afraid to get the demons out of your head using your own rituals that work for you. For me, going for a run or voicing my issues out loud is quite therapeutic. It may look strange to anyone who sees me in the process but it certainly works for me.

This is so much healthier compared to the demons rummaging around in your head and going over and over damaging thoughts.

Often, we don't know where these demons come from and you could spend years, the rest of your life even, trying to work that out. If you go down this path without professional help, it can be quite confusing, self-destructive and disempowering. I find it more empowering to take control of the demons and acknowledge them for what they are. They are not your reality and you are not defined by them. They are not you.

Acknowledging your demons is important because so often people allow themselves to be defined by something that has happened or a comment from the past. They ask, "Why is this happening to me?" I believe this is one of the most disempowering questions you can ask yourself. You need to say, "Okay, this has happened to me. What am I going to do about it? I'm complaining about this, so I need to acknowledge it."

As author and entrepreneur Jack Canfield said—"You only have control over three things in your life: the thoughts you think, the images you visualise, and the actions you take."

Ask yourself whether this is something you can control or change. You can only be in control of your intention and where you're investing your attention. You can then focus on what you actually want and what you're going to do about the situation.

Deliberately writing your goals and intentions out helps you focus your intentions and attention in a powerful way. In fact, as I mentioned earlier, research shows that writing your goals down makes you 42% more likely to achieve them than those who don't.[3] That's worth the repeat if you ask me.

Saying affirmations into a mirror or collating them onto a vision board can also act as great physical reminders. These are things you can control.

Some helpful affirmation to use are:
- My mind is powerful and strong
- I easily choose new and positive thoughts
- I liberate myself from fear, judgement and self-doubt
- Life brings me only good experiences
- I accept new and wonderful changes in my life
- I am at ease in my mind
- I choose the best and I deserve the best
- I release any negative past experiences easily and effortlessly
- I am in charge of my mind and body

Affirmations are powerful directives that communicate to your subconscious mind and build a strong mindset as long as you believe them.

Unfortunately, sometimes demons are stubborn and not going anywhere. Each time you're aiming for your next goal and worried you might fail, that inner critic will be there, lying in wait to start doubting yourself.

Once again, you need to put a timeframe on the amount of doubt you allow, acknowledging the mental demons and understanding what they're trying to do is a huge part of controlling them. Allow the demons their time limit and then begin thinking about indulging in your dreams. Returning to your affirmations and intentions set your mind for success.

The power is in your hands and you can choose which one is going to control you.

You may not know what the next step is in the process to reach your goals but allow yourself the space to visualise, imagine, dream and think of the exciting possibilities.

The more you do this, then that next step will appear, but only if you're listening.

PROCRASTINATION—A DOUBLE-EDGED SWORD

Procrastination can be a great tool if you know how to use it. Procrastinate on the mental demons and use them in a way that assists you towards where you want to go, as opposed to taking you away from your goal. It can be an absolutely fantastic tool to harness to use towards positive outcomes.

For example, I decide I'm going to procrastinate on my shitty, negative thinking for 5–10 minutes and then I'm going to focus on those other things that I know will take me towards achieving my goals. I give the negative thinking some time to be acknowledged but then I silence it and head in the direction of my dreams.

Procrastinating can also work against you and stop you achieving your goals. When you've made a plan to achieve something and you're not following through, it means you're not doing what you need to be doing. That's invalidating the agreement you have made with yourself. This will absolutely set off your inner critic because by violating that important personal vow you end up feeling frustrated with yourself.

You then need to either make a new agreement with yourself or decide to follow through on the original agreement. That's the only way out of that situation. I think it's also about being true to your word and not agreeing to something you know you can't, or won't follow through with.

If you find yourself in a situation where you're not going to follow through with something, renegotiate the agreement. Don't leave it in and then not do something about it. This applies to agreements with yourself and with other people.

ARE YOU HESITATING, PROCRASTINATING OR AVOIDING?

There is a difference between hesitation and procrastination. You can choose to hesitate or procrastinate.

Procrastination is putting stuff off and not following through on things.

Hesitation is when you're holding yourself back from doing something. Sometimes that can be for a good reason. There may be more information that you need in order to follow through. Or do you have enough of the information you need to go for it? Or, are you just hesitating because of fear?

Avoidance is something entirely different. When you're avoiding something, you're not wanting to look at it and you're not willing to confront a situation. For example, you've got a three-hundred-foot gorilla in the room and you want to pretend that it's not there. That's never going to work. Avoidance, as a tool, doesn't work.

Hesitation is a step forward from avoidance because at least you're willing to acknowledge the fear. But you just haven't fully worked through the information to deal with it.

Can you figure out which demon you're fighting? Is it avoidance? Or can you find a way to use procrastination to your advantage?

SILENCING MY WEIGHTLIFTING DEMONS

You can apply this technique to other aspects of life and do exactly the same thing—pause the conversation momentarily, acknowledge the thoughts because they are real but you've set up a protection mechanism to allow for some space and to counteract them.

When you watch professional elite athletes, they have a methodical process they go through to help them manage their inner critic and focus on the present. Keeping the mental negativity at bay is essential to success. Mental coach George Mumford, famous for helping famous basketballers such as Michael Jordan and Kobe Bryant get their mental edge, calls the demons of negative thinking and criticism—stinkin' thinkin'. Learning to control and eliminate stinkin' thinkin' is the key to success.

I personally use my own ritual when competing in weightlifting.

With Olympic weightlifting, when you're about to compete, go out on a platform and lift a weight above your head, you only have seconds to perform that action and for the weight not to come crashing down on your head. This means you can't let that voice, that shitty thinking, take over because that would be the worst thing.

When I'm preparing to lift more than my own bodyweight above my head, supported only by my physical strength, this is *not* the time to listen to my inner critic and start doubting myself. You simply don't have time to hesitate, but I did, with every competition.

My training taught me you can't have any thoughts going through your head, apart from the lift and the weight over your head. Silence is the best place to be. If there is chitter chatter happening in my head, I know I'm not going to perform well because this 'noise' is self-defeating. Thoughts like, *I don't know if I can do this, this is heavy, did I warm up enough? My toe hurts.* Even random thoughts like, *what did I have for breakfast?* Everything other than being present in the moment.

To counteract this chitter chatter, I would go through a ritual when I was chalking my hands before a lift, which is what you need to do. My mind would be going a million miles an hour with the adrenaline, but I would make sure I went through this ritual to silence the voice in my head. I would say to myself, *I pay gratitude and say thank you very much for your opinion, but right now I'm going to leave you at this chalk bowl. If I need you to, I can come back and I'll pick you up. But for now, I'm leaving you here.*

That ritual would then create the space I needed in my head to focus on the lift I would have this conversation in my head. It would allow me to pause the story and go and do what I needed to do.

By the time I came back to the chalkboard I had completely forgotten about whatever the heck was going on in my head and would follow that ritual for every competition.

But in life, we're typically so all over the shop that we don't have these methodical processes in place. As the adage says, "If you fail to plan, you plan to fail." So, I suggest to all my clients that they need to put something in place to help you handle your own chitter chatter and get in control.

For me, from a business point of view, when my mind races away from me, I just completely absorb myself in my favourite audiobooks and just keep listening to the messages they're giving me. I know I'll hear one key point from a podcast or an audiobook that helps me calm my mind down.

YOU BATTLE THE DEMONS WITH COURAGE, ACTION AND EFFORT

Just like I do when my mental demons start to get the better of me on a business front, it helps to take action in a positive direction. Trying and effort are your noble superpowers. They aren't to be underestimated. Effort, no matter how small, is an act of courage and it shows that you're willing to confront the demons head-on and not let them mess with you.

Dr Brené Brown became famous for encouraging people to be vulnerable and to dare greatly in life. To dare greatly involves a level of emotional vulnerability; for what if you try and fail, right? What if you use all your effort but don't win the prize?

But it's not the result that counts. It's the courageous effort that dispels the demons. It's the confrontation of them which silences them.

Former President of the United States, Theodore Roosevelt gave his famous "The Man in the Arena" speech at the Sorbonne in Paris, France, on April 23, 1910. It's been a source of inspiration for Brené's work and shows that it's the attitude that conquers one's mental demons. Although it uses male pronouns (it was back in 1910 remember)—it is relevant for anyone regardless of gender, age or culture.

"IT IS NOT THE CRITIC WHO COUNTS; NOT THE MAN WHO POINTS OUT HOW THE STRONG MAN STUMBLES, OR WHERE THE DOER OF DEEDS COULD HAVE DONE THEM BETTER. THE CREDIT BELONGS TO THE MAN WHO IS ACTUALLY IN THE ARENA, WHOSE FACE IS MARRED BY DUST AND SWEAT AND BLOOD; WHO STRIVES VALIANTLY; WHO ERRS, WHO COMES SHORT AGAIN AND AGAIN, BECAUSE THERE IS NO EFFORT WITHOUT ERROR AND SHORTCOMING; BUT WHO DOES ACTUALLY STRIVE TO DO THE DEEDS; WHO KNOWS GREAT ENTHUSIASMS, THE GREAT DEVOTIONS; WHO SPENDS HIMSELF IN A WORTHY CAUSE; WHO AT THE BEST KNOWS IN THE END THE TRIUMPH OF HIGH ACHIEVEMENT, AND WHO AT THE WORST, IF HE FAILS, AT LEAST FAILS WHILE DARING GREATLY, SO THAT HIS PLACE SHALL NEVER BE WITH THOSE COLD AND TIMID SOULS WHO NEITHER KNOW VICTORY NOR DEFEAT."[4]

I encourage you to take some time to think about the inner demons demanding your attention and the impact they're having on your life. Is there a recurring theme in your negative self-talk and how are you managing it?

Which one are you feeding? Here's a hint:

Dreams say:	Demons say:
I can do it	You will never do it
I am good enough	You're not good enough
I am capable of success	You'll never make it
I'm strong	You're weak
I deserve this	You don't deserve this
I can succeed	You will fail
I belong	You don't belong

Take action	Procrastinate and avoid
Make plans	Fail to plan
Affirm success	Deny success
Try with courage	Avoid trying from fear of failure
Encourage your potential	Criticise your plans
Encourage abundance	Tell you you're selfish
Control their mind.	Let their mind control them

UNLEASH YOUR MENTAL SUPERPOWERS

Your mind is your superpower. But it can also be your kryptonite if you don't use it properly.

The first step to unleashing your superpower is to **control the controllables.**

1. Define what you can control and what you can't.

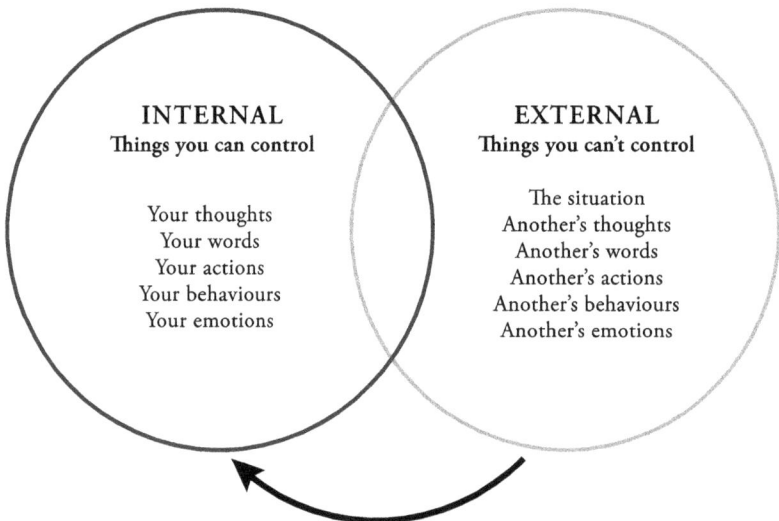

INTERNAL
Things you can control

Your thoughts
Your words
Your actions
Your behaviours
Your emotions

EXTERNAL
Things you can't control

The situation
Another's thoughts
Another's words
Another's actions
Another's behaviours
Another's emotions

How to control a situation?
Frame questions to yourself in terms of things you can control.
Move the centre of control of your focus from external to internal.

2. Focus your mind (through affirmations, visualisation, thoughts) on what you can control.

3. When the negative demons (thoughts of criticism, doubt, worry or judgement) arise, then give them a time limit. Indulge in them freely for a specified amount of time and then get up and do something else that is positive in the direction of your dreams.

4. Action heroes are heroes because they take action! Take immediate bold action towards your dreams.

Use the Reflect, Decide and Act prompts below to take control of your mind and banish those negatives that hold you back.

UNLEASHING YOUR SEVENTH SUPERPOWER
UNDERSTANDING AND MANAGING YOUR DEMONS

REFLECT

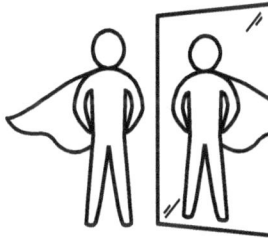

How many times throughout your day do you find yourself listening to your inner critic?

....

....

....

What is your inner critic telling you? How can you find evidence this is not true? Write down the critical statement and then find evidence to prove it inaccurate.

Example:

Inner critic says, *I'm not smart enough to be successful in business.*

Evidence that shows otherwise:

- I have succeeded at other things in life without knowing everything first.
- With good training and hard work many people have succeeded in business.
- Business is not an IQ test, it's about experience and effort and having good guidance.

Is this inner critic having an impact on you achieving your life goals? If so, how? How can you combat the inner critic's opinion?

Do you find yourself comparing yourself with other people? If so, how often?

What are you actually comparing? Looks, wealth, success? How does this make you feel?

....

....

....

....

....

....

What is an alternate story? Write down your new story without your inner critic in charge. How does life look without your inner critic centre stage?

....

....

....

....

....

....

....

....

....
....
....
....
....

What is an alternate story?

....
....
....
....
....
....
....
....
....
....
....
....
....
....

....

....

....

....

....

....

....

DECIDE

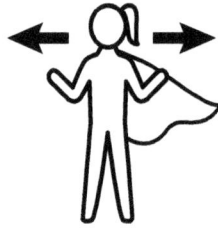

That you are going to be your own best friend.

That you're going to look after your basic needs, including eating well, exercising and getting plenty of sleep.

That you're going to do an audit of your social media and stop looking at things that make you feel bad about yourself and feed your inner critic.

That you're only going to surround yourself with people who build you up and help you achieve your dreams.

To develop a more empowering and accurate dialogue with yourself and stop the negative self-talk.

ACT

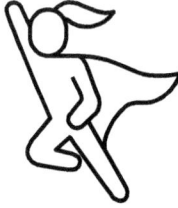

Make a conscious effort to stop critical self-talk before it spirals out of control. Set a timer.

Examine the evidence and learn to recognise when your critical thoughts are exaggeratedly negative.

Write down all the negative messages your demons are telling you then rip it up into tiny pieces. Burn the pieces of paper if you feel the need to.

Fill your fridge and pantry with healthy, nourishing food.

Schedule in at least one hour of outdoor exercise a day and start going to bed an hour early.

Limit your screen time and don't waste time on consuming media that feeds your demons.

Speak your affirmations regularly and perhaps even out loud.

Visualise your dreams and the next action you need to make towards it.

"

CALMNESS IS
A HUMAN
SUPERPOWER.
THE ABILITY
TO NOT OVERREACT
OR TAKE THINGS
PERSONALLY KEEPS
YOUR MIND
CLEAR AND
YOUR HEART
AT PEACE.

"

Marc and Angel Chernoff

The Shield of Immunity

"

GREATNESS BEGINS BEYOND YOUR COMFORT ZONE.

"

Robin Sharma

Purpose

Inside of you is your greatness, you may or may not be able to see this yet. Others may or may not be able to see this yet. As you journey through life allow yourself to follow the calling inside, those whispers, those dreams.

Take the time to dream and imagine again. This will build your immunity to all else that is occurring around you.

Check out Alison's personal video to you, the reader, about Superpower 8 in the bonus interactive book. Go to **deanpublishing.com/alisonwheeler** to discover more.

"

SISTERS IN BATTLE,
I AM SHIELD AND
BLADE TO YOU.
AS I BREATHE,
YOUR ENEMIES
WILL KNOW NO
SANCTUARY.
WHILE I LIVE YOUR
CAUSE IS MINE.

"

Wonder Woman: Warbringer

As you navigate life, I think it's important to be fully aware of both your strengths and weaknesses because this will give you a better understanding of who you really are and how you function.

Understanding your weaknesses gives you some insight into what's holding you back so you're better able to overcome them.

Identifying your strengths and understanding how they work, means you're able to use them to your full advantage.

Did you also know your weak points can actually turn out to be your strengths? I like to look upon them as a double-edged sword.

This is something I took many years to learn because I've always been a very driven and determined person. I also wanted to demonstrate this strength to the outside world, going to great lengths to hide any signs of weakness.

It was only when I reached the mid-stage of my life that I began to appreciate the importance of accepting my fragility, as well as my vulnerability. Owning my mistakes was all part of this.

As a result, I'm now more aware of my weak points and willing to admit them.

I think one of them is being overly critical and impatient, mainly towards myself. If I'm having a particularly bad day it can reflect over into my relationship with others as well.

Because I'm naturally impatient, I like things to happen quickly and if people don't work according to my timeframe, I tend to get frustrated. That can be challenging.

As a result, over the years I've had to learn to interact with the world and accept not everyone operates at the level I do, and that's okay.

There are so many aspects of our lives that represent a double-edged sword. But just as a sword has two sides, everything considered a weakness may also represent a strength.

For example, I tend to over-think and reflect on things deeply, which I think represents another double-edged sword.

On the one hand, this may be considered a strength as being self-aware can have several advantages. On the other hand, it may also be considered a weakness. Ruminating too much can lead to anxiety and depression.

Because I'm impatient and love testing the boundaries, it means I get a lot of things done. That's my strength. On the other hand, sometimes I don't recognise when I've pushed myself too far and come dangerously close to burnout. I guess that's my weakness.

There is often a very fine line between your strengths and weaknesses, particularly if you want to perform at the highest level and fully express yourself. Think of many great creative artists, they are borderline genius with their self-expression and uniqueness, yet many find this same strength can make them feel lonely and isolated and lead to drug dependency or an inability to connect with others.

Being aware of and understanding your strengths and weaknesses will help you identify where this fine line is.

FULL EXPRESSION

You can turn your weak points into strengths by owning and understanding them, as well as accepting that you don't have to be strong in every single area.

It's okay to have areas you're not strong at because you will always find people who can help fill in the gaps and support you.

For example, I would rather have someone cleaning my house because for me it's not something I enjoy doing, nor is it a priority for me. There are other things I'd much rather be doing.

This means accepting there are only so many hours in the day and that there's nothing wrong with delegating time-consuming tasks, like housework, to other people.

If you believe you're 'super-human' and able to do everything on your own, you're not being truthful with yourself and this will gradually chip away at your power. Each time you do that, you diminish yourself and become a little less powerful.

Similarly, if you make a mistake but you don't acknowledge it, you risk losing the respect of others and yourself.

For example, anyone who has children knows that parenting is one of the toughest jobs there is and it's important to remind ourselves that we're human and that there will be good days and bad days.

Sometimes things don't go how I intend in my relationship with my daughter and I react the wrong way. I could pretend it didn't happen and sweep it under the carpet, or, alternatively, go back to my daughter and say, "Look, I handled that really poorly. I'm really sorry about that. Can we have another go?"

This is an important lesson for children because it teaches them the importance of honesty, that adults aren't always perfect and can make mistakes. They also learn they don't have to be invincible and that mistakes are okay because you can fix them, or at least have another try.

CRAZY BREADCRUMB IDEAS

When we go after a goal and we change it into a game rather than something to conquer, we can lighten the load and aspire to something new or great, or bigger, or better, without the demands attached.

As we think about our new game and how we're going to achieve it, we can often get some new and crazy ideas. I think these ideas actually come from your true self, and often many of these crazy ideas don't seem to be a part of your normal way of being. These are the crazy, breadcrumb, hare-brained ideas. I've learned these are the ideas you need to follow to succeed.

Everyone is capable of coming up with crazy ideas but sometimes these ideas seem so crazy, we're almost too embarrassed to share them with others and dismiss them as unrealistic. However, crazy ideas can often lead to the most interesting insights. You may even be able to turn a crazy idea into a feasible idea. This is because crazy breadcrumb ideas can be used as stepping-stones to generate creative, workable ideas.

To turn the idea into something workable you just need to ask yourself three things:

- What value does this idea contain?
- What are the cons to this idea?
- What are the main principles behind this idea?
- When you're going after a goal and thinking about how you're going

to achieve it, make sure you don't ignore those crazy ideas that tend to pop in your head because they are all part of the game.

These are the ideas that pop in your head and you think—*Oh, that's totally ridiculous I can't do that!* These are exactly the ideas you need to follow.

Will this idea pan out in exactly what you want it to? Maybe, maybe not, who knows? But by listening to and following them, you'll be a lot closer to the next part of the puzzle being revealed.

I think these ideas are actually coming from your true self even though they may not seem logical or part of your normal way of being. There is a saying that it's easier to 'tame' a wild idea than it is to make a dull idea look interesting. I think this is why Steve Jobs quote is so loved—

> *"HERE'S TO THE CRAZY ONES. THE MISFITS. THE REBELS. THE TROUBLEMAKERS. THE ROUND PEGS IN THE SQUARE HOLES. THE ONES WHO SEE THINGS DIFFERENTLY. THEY'RE NOT FOND OF RULES. AND THEY HAVE NO RESPECT FOR THE STATUS QUO. YOU CAN QUOTE THEM, DISAGREE WITH THEM, GLORIFY OR VILIFY THEM. ABOUT THE ONLY THING YOU CAN'T DO IS IGNORE THEM. BECAUSE THEY CHANGE THINGS. THEY PUSH THE HUMAN RACE FORWARD. AND WHILE SOME MAY SEE THEM AS THE CRAZY ONES, WE SEE GENIUS. BECAUSE THE PEOPLE WHO ARE CRAZY ENOUGH TO THINK THEY CAN CHANGE THE WORLD, ARE THE ONES WHO DO."*
>
> ***STEVE JOBS – APPLE INC.***

In fact, did you know some of the most famous world-changing inventions that we take for granted today, were initially ridiculed and rejected, including:

- The electric lightbulb
- The telephone
- The television
- Personal computers
- The photocopier
- Vaccines

- Aeroplanes
- Cars

Even the humble bicycle was ridiculed and called a passing fad. Experts published a statement about bicycles in the *Washington Post* saying "the popularity of the wheel is doomed." Can you imagine that?

Laptops were also publicly reported to be "on their way out" and even talking in films was considered a passing trend. The President of United Artists, Joseph Schenck openly declared to the *New York Times* that "talking doesn't belong in pictures." When asked about talking, he said, "I don't think people will want talking pictures long."

Needless to say, the bikes and the talking films are now such a part of our daily lives we wouldn't consider them once radical or extreme ideas at all.

The list of so-called crazy ideas that changed our world is long. In fact, we have built our world with these ideas. We changed the landscape of what is possible simply because a small group of people decided to take their ideas seriously. I can't help but admire these pioneering people, the ones who didn't play small or let self-doubt and criticism stop their dreams from coming true.

As Elon Musk said, "Good ideas are always crazy until they are not."

BODYBUILDING

I like to think of getting started with bodybuilding as perhaps one of my craziest breadcrumb ideas yet.

I knew I wanted to be more self-expressed and reach the next level in my business as well as improve my health and then bodybuilding came into my reality. At the time, I remember thinking, *seriously this is ridiculous.* I knew I had to give up a lot of other stuff and change a whole lot of things in order to follow through with bodybuilding. But I thought—*Well hold on a second. How do I know this is not the very thing I need to do? This is what's been delivered. I at least deserve to investigate it thoroughly. Because what if that is exactly the answer that I've been looking for? And unless I investigate that, I will never know.*

I've had this same experience with all sorts of other ideas I've had when people have challenged me and asked, "Why do you want to do that?"

That then led to my own internal battle where I began to question these crazy ideas and whether or not to follow them.

I then realised these crazy ideas of mine were popping into my head for a reason—to unlock me and give me the freedom to make my own decisions. To explore, to grow, to be me.

If you have your own crazy ideas, it's important to remember they are your ideas and belong to no-one else.

They are your answer to the question about what you need to do to achieve your goals. Every single idea you have is an expression of you and the choice you have is to either ignore them or follow through with them.

When I'm coaching, I encourage my clients to listen to their crazy breadcrumb ideas—identify them, write them down, and then think about how they can follow through with them.

Often the people I coach have so much potential but are full of fear. They have big goals but then 'imposter syndrome' kicks in—They doubt their abilities and feel like a fraud. They're afraid someone may challenge them and ridicule their 'crazy' idea.

I let my clients know that this feeling is not uncommon and that it's a matter of acknowledging it for what it is and building faith along the way.

I've successfully applied this strategy in our business and recommend it if you're starting out or wanting to expand your business. As my husband knows all too well, I am constantly coming up with crazy ideas to expand our business. It could be a marketing idea, or I'd google something and say to my husband, "Let's try this!"

Sometimes when I have these ideas I'll be nowhere near where I can write them down, such as in the shower or at yoga, or I wake up in the middle of the night with an idea in my head. I now make sure I have some way of recording each time an idea comes into my head, especially when I don't have pen and paper handy. I often use voice memo notes on my phone which now has so many notes on it of the ideas I've documented and want to come back to

Sometimes there may be notes I don't need, or use, but they just lead to the next thing. Amongst all these ideas, some of them were actually going to work and the idea is to follow through with them as fast as possible and see what the outcome is.

Will these ideas pan out into exactly what you want them to be? Maybe, maybe not. Who knows?

But what I do know is that you're going to be a hell of a lot closer than you were by following these ideas because the next thing will be revealed when you listen to them, and then the next.

UNLEASHING YOUR EIGHT SUPERPOWER
LISTENING TO AND VALUING YOUR CRAZY IDEAS

REFLECT

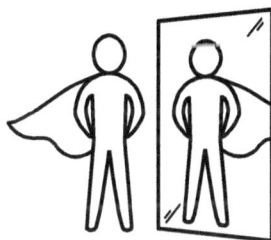

When and where do you find yourself coming up with unique and creative, perhaps slightly crazy ideas? Perhaps it's when you're in a certain place or doing a mundane activity, such as driving or the washing up?

What do you do with these ideas?

....

....

....

....

....

....

....

....

....

....

List some of your best and craziest ideas?

....

....

....

....

....

....

....

....

....

....

....

....

....

....

....

....

....

....

....

....

....

DECIDE

To give yourself time and space each day to think and perhaps even daydream.

To allow ideas to flow into your mind and listen to them.

ACT

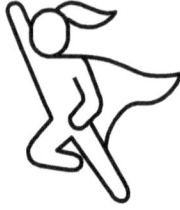

Each day write down five ideas that pop into your head, no matter how crazy and random they may seem.

List your first five crazy ideas for the day/week.

1. ....

....

2. ....

....

3. ....

....

4. ....

....

5. ....

....

Take one of these crazy ideas and write down the steps you think you'll need to follow to bring it to fruition.

Steps I need to take are:

....

....

....

....

....

....

....

....

....

....

....

....

....

....

....

....

....

....

....

"

MY ATTITUDE
IS IF YOU PUSH
ME TOWARDS
SOMETHING THAT
YOU THINK IS
A WEAKNESS,
THEN I WILL TURN
THAT PERCEIVED
WEAKNESS INTO
A STRENGTH.

"

Michael Jordan

The Battlefield

"

LIFE IS JUST
LIKE A GAME,
FIRST YOU HAVE
TO LEARN RULES
OF THE GAME,
AND THEN PLAY
IT BETTER THEN
ANY ONE ELSE.

"

Albert Einstein

Purpose

This chapter is to bring it all together.
You are ready. It is time to step up to
the game of life and live fully as you.
Life is a game and you get to play it, you
can decide on the rules, the playing field,
the opponents and the prize.

What is your game going to be?

Check out Alison's personal video to
you, the reader, about Superpower 9
in the bonus interactive book. Go to
deanpublishing.com/alisonwheeler
to discover more.

"

WE WORK TO HAVE LEISURE— ON WHICH HAPPINESS DEPENDS.

"

Aristotle

I used to treat my life for a very long time as if it was a battle. It was me in the world universe up against someone else—God, creator, a higher power, whatever you want to call it.

But this was not how I wanted it. It didn't feel right. It felt like something was missing.

It was this constant battle where I always felt on the defensive, or the offensive. I felt like a stoic warrior, constantly prepared to go into battle.

When you go through life feeling as though you have to be a warrior, you are going to miss a lot of important experiences because you're always on the defensive.

If you're in a constant state of fight or flight you're not tapping into that part of your brain that allows you to see the beauty in the world, or those moments when you just need to stop and catch your breath.

I eventually came to the realisation that I didn't always need to approach life as a competition, or some sort of battle. I needed to stop the battle, but it's no good stopping something unless you have something to put in its place. This is because you end up picking up the same thing and falling back into the same bad habits.

So, for me it was creating a game, like we do with children when we ask them to tidy their rooms. You can nag and plead, and that battle can go on endlessly. Or, you can make it into a game and say, *"Okay. Let's see if you can tidy your room in five minutes,"* and turn it into a game. You'll find kids will put a whole lot of energy into it and then all of sudden the room is tidy.

I tend to use this strategy all the time with my daughter. I also use it with myself and test myself to just see what I can actually achieve. How do I know what I can do if I don't test it out and see what's possible?

Injecting fun into things and seeing what I can achieve in ten minutes, for example, stops me taking life too seriously and seeing what's possible. You can use the same game when it comes to the bigger picture and seeing what's possible to achieve in life.

Once you begin to challenge the entrenched attitudes and social expectations, we all deal with, you can actually start approaching life as a game.

To do this you really need to start listening to those crazy breadcrumb ideas that pop into your head at inopportune times. Those spark of ideas I spoke about in the previous chapter. These are the keys to liberating your true self and allowing yourself to be fully expressed and achieve your goals.

So, why do we feel we need to approach life as a battle, or as a competition?

I believe we are indoctrinated into that way of thinking through what we learn at school and by the media we consume which tends to encourage competition, fear and rage.

Everywhere, we see examples of people fighting against each other to be right. People are constantly engaging in hurtful and sometimes destructive arguments via social media.

Our politicians are constantly engaged in battle and countless pointless wars have been fought around the world with tragic human losses. Half the time, at the end of it all, the countries fighting each other don't even know what it's all about.

If you want to stop treating life as a battlefield and more as a game, you need to consider other peoples' points of view and agree to disagree.

You also need to stop battling against life and against yourself. That is equally as important.

Admittedly, many things in life are set up as a competition and I don't necessarily think there's anything wrong with having winners and losers. After all, life doesn't give you a gold medal for just turning up.

However, that doesn't necessarily mean you're in competition with everyone else because, at the end of the day, the only person you're in competition with is yourself.

It's your game but you need to move from a competitive state, where you're constantly engaged in a win/lose situation and adopt a different approach.

It's not about who wins or loses. It's about learning and developing as a person.

If you take this approach it means you can engage in a game which is much more light-hearted and a hell of a lot more fun!

The game may still have all the same trappings as a competition but there are rules and boundaries which you can navigate around so much more easily.

On the other hand, if you're engaged in a battle, you're constantly ready to fight and this is where your focus is. There's only one stance and that's fight or be killed. That means you're unable to focus on the positive aspects of life and the vision you have for it.

WHAT'S YOUR GAME?

If you approach life as a game, it means you'll find yourself constantly navigating and negotiating, contemplating your next move—like a puzzle game that involves moving the pieces and doing what you need to do to achieve the winning outcome.

When you think back to your childhood and how much you learnt through simple play, you begin to understand how powerful this approach can be.

I've applied this approach in business a lot. I've had people who want to compete with me, I don't want to compete with you. *Stay in your own lane my friend.*

There might be a winner and loser in this situation, obviously. But I'm not in competition with other people. I'm in competition with myself.

The 'game' for me involves looking at the goal I want to achieve. I think about the outcome I'm looking for and what's involved. I think to myself, *what are all the puzzle pieces and how do they all fit in?*

How can I move the next puzzle piece in order to get closer to that outcome? What seems like the most logical next step? And I just keep looking for the next puzzle piece to move. When the next idea comes into my head, I follow through with that, particularly when I'm really going after a goal.

Sometimes, they don't seem like they fit it, but this idea has come to me for a reason, because it's part of that game and so I follow through with that. This approach has allowed me to achieve some huge goals in my business.

I had my most recent goal of 200,000 US dollars profit in one month in business. I did that by applying the 'puzzle strategy'. I just looked for the next puzzle piece to move in order to keep in constant flow. If I felt it slowing down, I would say, *okay, now I need to move another puzzle piece. What is that? What is that going to be?* I didn't know so I just waited.

It's important to be focused on your own game and your own strategy and not engage in conflict or someone else's battle.

Looking outside of yourself, at what everyone else is doing can be such a massive distraction and often takes people out of the game because they're comparing themselves to others.

This is particularly relevant when it comes to social media because people only post their best pictures. They're portraying this perfect life, but what's really going on in the background? They could be one pay cheque away from being bankrupt or in a toxic relationship that disempowers them. You just don't know when it's all nice and shiny on the outside.

This means you fall into the trap of competing and comparing, instead of focusing on and following your own path. This can create so much unhappiness and dissatisfaction because you end up chasing the wrong game—you're chasing an unattainable goal based on a fictional idea. Or even worse, you are chasing someone else's goal.

This is a disempowering way to live and results in a loss of personal power because you're no longer playing your game—you're no longer the mastermind moving the puzzle pieces.

If you're waiting for someone else to give you the green light, you're playing their game, not yours. You're not even in your own game. You are literally sitting on the sideline watching.

When you feel you have to wait for permission before you can play your own game you become a sideline contender—an observer of your life, not doing what you need to do to learn the lessons to make the next move.

You are the only one who can give yourself the green light for the next move. However, so often we wait for permission from someone else and then we start making excuses and procrastination creeps in.

When this happens, you have to remember that this is your goal, so you have to take responsibility for it, as well as the outcomes.

For example, if my husband and I haven't proven ourselves in a particular area of our business, this does not mean that we don't move forward in that area. If it happens to be my idea to pursue a new business idea, then I can acknowledge my husband's concerns and hesitation, but ultimately the onus is on *me* to work towards that goal, and vice versa.

Interestingly, big business has also discovered that treating life as a game can be highly profitable.

A consumer trend called 'gamification,' where video games and other devices take real life situations and incorporate features such as missions, scoring, rewards, badges and ranks, has become increasingly popular.

According to forecasts, the global gamification market is expected to grow from 4.9 billion US dollars in 2016, to nearly 12 billion in 2021.[1]

There is also increasing evidence that incorporating 'play' into your routine is a fantastic way to combine learning with daily life. Research shows that it not only clarifies the theoretical concepts in a tangible way, but it strengthens your mind/body connection which experts have shown is essential to success.

There's even scientific research to suggest that playing games can actually increase your lifespan.

American author and world-renowned games designer, Jane McGonigal, saw the potential in 'play' to improve real lives and solve real problems.

In 2009, Jane suffered a serious concussion and was unable to think clearly, or even get out of bed, she became anxious and depressed, to the point of being suicidal. Not to be broken, Jayne turned her recovery and rehab into a resilience-building game and started to use simple motivational exercises to help her recover. Using these resilience-building rules led her to design a digital game, SuperBetter, and embark on a major research study with the National Institute of Health.[2]

Decades of scientific research shows that video games, sports and puzzles change how we respond to stress, challenges and pain. Simply by adopting a more playful mindset, this research demonstrated how we can cultivate new powers of recovery and resilience in everyday life.

A new app called MoodMission even gives you five simple and effective, evidence-based 'Missions' to improve your mood if you're suffering from anxiety, depression or low moods. They are designed through scientific evidence to boost mental health and happiness.

For those wanting something a little different, there are funny apps to gamify simple tasks like doing chores or building habits. For example, ChoreWars allows roommates or family members to compete and keep score of who does the chores. Or for those who want to make their exercise experience very different—there's Zombies, Run! An app where you are given a mission and are chased by zombies in order to get some exercise. Now, I personally don't need zombies to help me exercise, but the point is you can be creative in the way you go about your day. It doesn't have to be 'normal' or what other people do; you can live your life out-of-the-box if you want to.

GAMES ARE A MENTAL SUPERPOWER

Being playful means bringing the same psychological strengths we naturally display when we play games, such as optimism and creativity as well as courage and determination to achieve real world goals.

Playing games taps into three core psychological strengths that help you build:

- Your ability to help you control your attention and therefore your thoughts and feelings
- Your power to turn anyone into a potential ally and to strengthen your existing relationships
- Your natural capacity to motivate yourself and supercharge your heroic qualities, such as willpower, compassion and determination

Approaching a challenging task as a game also makes it easier as it encourages you to break goals down into levelled steps.

One man who took his life to the next level and made it one big adventure is owner of the business Nerd Fitness, Steve Kamb. Steven gamified his life and transformed himself from a self-proclaimed daydreamer to a real-life superhero. Yes, he turned his life into a gigantic video game and reaped the rewards big time. His bestselling book *Level Up Your Life: How to Unlock Adventure and Happiness by Becoming the Hero of Your Own Story* showcases how he gave himself missions, earned points and even built systems and quests to help him level up his life.

Now, I'm not suggesting you need to be extreme and take on a whole new alter ego in order to make your life work, what I am suggesting is that you inject some fun and adventure into your life! To make it playful and full of laughs and wins and not just a never-ending to-do list.

You are worth the adventure! You are worth the fun and the joy!

Your life isn't here just for accomplishment and awards, it's here to be enjoyed and lived.

> "MOST PEOPLE CONSIDER LIFE A BATTLE,
> BUT IT IS NOT A BATTLE, IT IS A GAME."
> **FLORENCE SCOVEL SHINN,**
> **THE GAME OF LIFE AND HOW TO PLAY IT**

UNLEASHING YOUR NINTH SUPERPOWER
DEVELOPING A PLAYFUL MINDSET

REFLECT

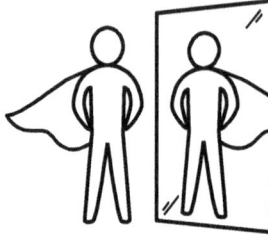

How do you see your life? As a battlefield or as a playground?

Think about how you approach challenges? Where is your focus?

Are you competing with yourself or with others?

DECIDE

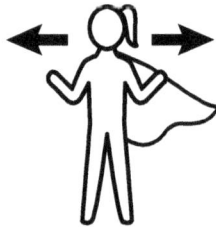

To undergo a 'digital detox,' in particular, take a break from all social media.

To try new things and experience the unexpected.

To appreciate playtime—whether it's alone, with children or other adults.

To create a happy, joyful, positive attitude, full of gratitude for even the smallest, everyday things.

ACT

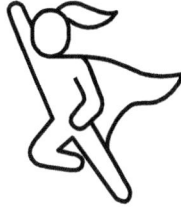

Sing and dance for the fun of it.

Decide to smile and laugh more often throughout the day.

Use unscheduled time to be creative, to daydream, reflect and decompress.

Spend as much time as possible with the children in your life, listen carefully to them and follow their train of thought.

List some ways you can bring play and fun into your daily life.

....

....

....

....

....

....

....

Epilogue

Now that you have made it to the end of the book, I'd like to suggest that this isn't an ending for you but a beginning. A new beginning for you to live your best life physically, mentally, emotionally and spiritually. For you to step out of self-doubt, self-neglect and self-sabotage and claim the life you were born to live.

Of course it can begin with a decision, and it gains momentum when you act on that decision.

As you've seen from my story, you don't have to be totally complete and perfect in order to take a first step; you just need to muster a tiny bit of courage to begin. The great champion boxer Muhammad Ali said, "Even the greatest was once a beginner. Don't be afraid to take that first step."

Living From the Inside-Out: How to Become a Modern-day Wonder Woman was written with you in mind. It was written to show you that with a few mindset shifts and a new way of looking at yourself, you can achieve things you never thought possible. How do I know this? Because as you've read, this was the same transformational journey I had to make to find my inner Wonder Woman and express myself fully in the world. It was one of the best decisions of my life.

A modern-day Wonder Woman can be and do many things. She can:

- Be vulnerable and strong at the same time.
- Prioritise self-care without guilt or shame.
- Make her own decisions and take responsibility for the outcome.
- Have a good relationship with herself and others.
- Live, work and play on her own terms.
- Be physically, emotionally and spiritually nourished in her daily life.
- Love herself and others fully.
- Rid herself of toxic relationships and environments.
- Live without seeking approval and permission from others.
- Stand up for herself and stand by her values.
- Have fun and play the game of life with a light heart.
- Be a role model for others.

You are this woman! And even if it doesn't feel like you right now, underneath your busy schedule, to-do lists, and never-ending cycle of caring for others, is a gorgeous being that is ready to express herself and become all she can be.

Now, I know that doing this alone can be daunting. I know that inside of you is your true self just busting to be free and live fearlessly. I have met so many women who feel the pulse of their potential inside and just need some help to break free.

My mission in life is to help you break free. To help you remove the shackles so you can dance freely and be all you're meant to be.

Of course, as a life coach, I won't do all the work for you, but I can certainly help you avoid the common pitfalls and encourage you out of your comfort zone and into your growth zone. I can cheer on your achievements and guide you towards the path of success and wellbeing.

Have you ever heard about the butterfly's need to struggle from the cocoon?

Well, let me tell you that there is great wisdom in their need to break open their own cocoon. You see, butterflies go through an incredible transformation, as they go from caterpillar to chrysalis to butterfly—they go through a process called metamorphosis. The definition of metamorphosis is a "change of physical form, structure, or substance especially by supernatural means."[1]

Essentially, butterflies transform from the inside-out. And in order to create wings and fly, they must go through the dark stage of the cocoon and the messy process of metamorphosis. They cannot become a beautiful butterfly without those processes.

And when it's time to break free and spread their wings, they must struggle! Why? Because when it's time for them to push their body through the small opening of the cocoon, the struggle causes specific fluid and hormones to flood their body and wings and give them the strength to fly. Without the struggle, butterflies would die and never fly.

I believe we are similar in many ways. We can also use our struggles to develop our wings and fly. Not by avoiding struggle, but by using our struggles to get airborne and reach great heights.

Once we have taken to the skies, we can see the whole panoramic view of life and access the big picture that was never available to us whilst in the darkness of the cocoon. When you have wings, you have full vision available to you. You can see further and longer than ever before.

I believe everyone is born with the capacity to reach their full potential, and the struggles and obstacles we face are to propel us higher, not to keep us down. Just like aeroplanes need the resistance of the wind in order to be lifted into the sky, we need resistance in order to become resilient.

Challenges do not define us, our ability to overcome them does. We aren't here to stay stagnant, we are here to grow and evolve. We are beings of transformation.

As you read, I finally made it through the other side, but it wasn't a straight and easy road. It was curvy and colourful. I believe that we all have our own journey, and it helps to walk the path with someone who has been there and done that. It doesn't mean that the paths are the same, it just means that you have someone alongside you that understands your wild adventure.

As the saying goes—*you didn't come this far to only come this far.* So, the question is: what next?

If you'd like to connect with me and take the next step to becoming your own version of a modern-day Wonder Woman, then please get in touch. I love living my best life with people who want to do the same. Let's take the journey together.

Alison

Alison is sharing more in her INTERACTIVE book.

See exclusive downloads, videos, audios and photos.

DOWNLOAD it for free at
deanpublishing.com/alisonwheeler

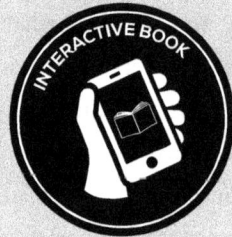

About The Author

Alison Wheeler is a true powerhouse in life and business. She is a multi-disciplined, award-winning performance athlete and celebrated entrepreneur. Having competed nationally in Olympic weightlifting, as well as rowing, CrossFit, athletics and bodybuilding, she has won multiple awards for her home country of New Zealand. Alison and her family now call the Gold Coast, Queensland home.

Ali is a celebrated businesswoman who has won multiple industry awards. Her success as an athlete and entrepreneur is magnetic, and her presence is real, raw and authentic.

But life hasn't always been easy for her. She suffered some significant health issues, and just when Ali could have let critical health issues stop her in her tracks, her determination kicked in. Ali's desire for a healthier body, loving relationships and a life beyond the

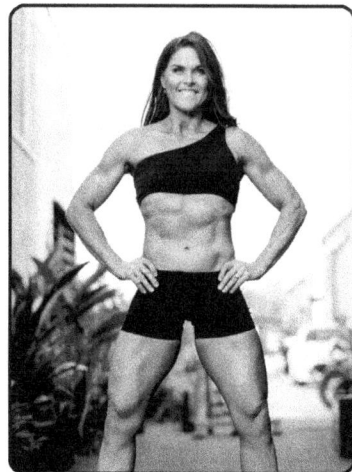

average led her to a place where she can impact the lives of others. Having focus, combined with the right balance of patience and persistence, and a whole lot of life experience, helps Alison give her clients the best. They often achieve things they once only dreamt about.

Alison's guidance helps her clients stretch themselves and reach their potential at a pace that sparks motivation and increases satisfaction. Even if they hit an obstacle, Ali helps them leap over it and learn to be and do their best on the other side. Alison is a published author, contributor and mentor. Her qualifications include a Bachelor of Health Science, NLP training, and many coaching certificates in a multitude of different practises.

She is passionate about helping women find their voice, reconnect with the goddess within, release the shame and guilt resulting from years of suppression and step into their true selves to find their freedom.

Alison loves empowering others to find their wisdom, truth, and inner Wonder Woman.

thealisonwheeler.com

Acknowledgements

I would like to thank the many people who have made a huge impact on my life and helped me become the person I am. You have all inspired me to voice the messages I am sharing.

To my dearest husband Paul: you are my rock and support. You see the best in me even when I can't. Without you I would not have completed this book or found my voice and started to share it more with the world. I am forever grateful to call you my husband and best friend.

To my daughter Jasmine, you are a shining star of pure love and joy in my life. You allow me to stay grounded in play and fun and the lightness of life, particularly when I get stuck in "work" mode. You are a beautiful young woman.

To my mum, and sisters and my dad (even though you are no longer with us), thank you for being the very best family to have been raised in. I always felt like I had the space to explore life and see what was possible.

To my coaching and business clients—you are all sensational. You push the boundaries of success and live fully. You are learning and growing always and holding me to the highest standards, inspiring me to lead by example.

To Susan and the Dean Publishing team: your support and dedication has been amazing, and I cannot thank you enough.

To my coaches and support team in business and my athletic life—thank you for always showing me the path forward, giving me the space to find my way and being there to catch me should I fall. You are a sounding board and inspiration.

To my modern-day Wonder Woman tribe: you are all amazing. You are successful and brilliant in all your real rawness. I have had the pleasure of working with each and every one of you and I have been moved. You teach me so much more than I could ever give to you. What an inspiration you all are.

Check out Alison's personal Thank You video @ **deanpublishing.com/ alisonwheeler**

Testimonials

"I feel incredibly grateful to have been mentored and coached by Alison over the last 11 years. Alison has helped and empowered me with several major life transitions, and I am so appreciative that we crossed paths so many years ago."

— **Carrie,** Mum, carer and coach

"I am forever grateful for this beautiful woman who is authentic and so passionate about sharing her struggles and insecurities…instead of seeing them as a sign of weakness, her vulnerability is her superpower."

— **Karen Murphy,** CEO and business owner

"Alison has inspired me both personally and professionally, she leads by example and has empowered me to live my best life!"

— **Natasha,** Mum and business owner

Endnotes

INTRODUCTION

1 Patanjali, *Yoga Sutras ("Method of Enlightenment,"* ca. Second Century B.C.)

SUPERPOWER 1

1 Brown, B 2018, *Dare to Lead: Brave Work. Tough Conversations. Whole Hearts.*, Random House, New York.

2 Katty, K & Shipman, C 2014, *The Confidence Code: The Science and Art of Self-Assurance - What Women Should Know,* HarperCollins, New York.

3 Mund, M., & Mitte, K. (2012). The costs of repression: A meta-analysis on the relation between repressive coping and somatic diseases. *Health Psychology*, 31(5), 640–649. https://doi.org/10.1037/a0026257

Mund, M., & Mitte, K. (2012). The costs of repression: A meta-analysis on the relation between repressive coping and somatic diseases. *Health Psychology*, 31(5), 640–649. https://doi.org/10.1037/a0026257

SUPERPOWER 2

1 Under the influence of the Lasso of Truth, Wonder Woman admits to herself the complex and powerful individual she is and realises that forces had been working against her to keep her from learning her own true history.

2 Aldosarri, M & Chaudhry, S 2020, 'Women and burnout in the context of a pandemic', *Feminist Frontiers*, vol 28, no 2, pp 826-834, https://onlinelibrary.wiley.com/doi/10.1111/gwao.12567#gwao12567-sec-0020-title

Purvanova, RK & Muros, JP 2010, 'Gender differences in burnout: A meta-analysis', *Journal of Vocational Behaviour*, vol 72, no 2, pp 168-185, https://www.researchgate.net/publication/229389297_Gender_differences_in_burnout_A_meta-analysis

3 Gerzema, J & D'Antonio, M 2013, *The Athena Doctrine: How Women (and the Men Who Think Like Them) Will Rule the Future*, Jossey-Bass, San Francisco.

4 Swan, Teal. https://tealswan.com/resources/articles/divine-feminine-vs-divine-masculine

5 Tamlin S. Conner, Colin G. DeYoung & Paul J. Silvia (2018) 'Everyday creative activity as a path to flourishing', The Journal of Positive Psychology, 13:2, 181-189, DOI: 10.1080/17439760.2016.1257049

6 Girija Kaimal, Hasan Ayaz, Joanna Herres, Rebekka Dieterich-Hartwell, Bindal Makwana, Donna H. Kaiser, Jennifer A. Nasser, 'Functional near-infrared spectroscopy assessment of reward perception based on visual self-expression: Coloring, doodling, and free drawing', The Arts in Psychotherapy, Volume 55, 2017, https://doi.org/10.1016/j.aip.2017.05.004

SUPERPOWER 3

1   Kamins, M. L., & Dweck, C. S. (1999). Person versus process praise and criticism: Implications for contingent self-worth and coping. *Developmental Psychology*, 35(3), 835–847. https://doi.org/10.1037/0012-1649.35.3.835

2   *Webster's New World College Dictionary*, 4th Edition, Houghton Mifflin Harcourt.

3   Zenger, Jack. Folkman, Joseph. Harvard Business Review, 'The Skills Leaders Need at Every Level', July 30, 2014, accessed online April 22, 2022.

SUPERPOWER 4

1   Sheldon, K. M. (2002). "The self-concordance model of healthy goal striving: when personal goals correctly represent the person" in *Handbook of self-determination research*. eds. E. L. Deci and R. M. Ryan (Rochester, NY: The University of Rochester Press), 65–86.

2   Nix, G. A., Ryan, R. M., Manly, J. B., and Deci, L. (1999). Revitalization through self-regulation: the effects of autonomous and controlled motivation on happiness and vitality. *J. Exp. Soc. Psychol.* 35, 266–284. doi: 10.1006/jesp.1999.1382

3   McGregor, I., and Little, B. R. (1998). Personal projects, happiness, and meaning: on doing well and being yourself. *J. Pers. Soc. Psychol.* 74, 494–512. doi: 10.1037/0022-3514.74.2.494

4   Sheldon, K. M., and Kasser, T. (1998). Pursuing personal goals: skills enable progress, but not all progress is beneficial. *Personal. Soc. Psychol. Bull.* 24, 1319–1331. doi: 10.1177/01461672982412006

5   Nurra, C., & Oyserman, D. (2018). From future self to current action: An identity-based motivation perspective. *Self and Identity, 17*(3), 343–364. https://doi.org/10.1080/15298868.2017.1375003

6   Branson, R 2005, *Losing My Virginity, The Autobiography*, Random House, Milsons Point, NSW.

7   Matthews, G, 2020, Goals Research Summary, PDF, Dominican University of California, California

8   Economy Peter, *Inc.* 28 Feb 2018, "This Is the Way You Need to Write Down Your Goals for Faster Success." Accessed July 15, https://www.inc.com/peter-economy/this-is-way-you-need-to-write-down-your-goals-for-faster-success.html

9   Green Carmichael, Sarah. August 19 2015, *Harvard Business Review*, Human Resource Management, "The Research Is Clear: Long Hours Backfire for People and for Companies." https://hbr.org/2015/08/the-research-is-clear-long-hours-backfire-for-people-and-for-companies

10 Ryan, E. D., & Simons, J. (1982). Efficacy of mental imagery in enhancing mental rehearsal of motor skills. *Journal of Sport Psychology, 4*, 41-51.

11 Covey, S 1989, *The 7 Habits of Highly Effective People*, Free Press, New York.

SUPERPOWER 5

1   Tracy, B 2011, *No Excuses! The Power of Self Discipline*, Little Brown and Company, Boston.

2   Nierenberg, C 2016, *The Science of Intuition: How to measure 'hunches' and 'gut feelings'*, webpage, Live Science, https://www.livescience.com/54825-scientists-measure-intuition.html

SUPERPOWER 6

1   ECMC Group 2021, *Generation Z Career Plans and Expectations*, webpage, ECMC Group, Minneapolis, https://www.ecmcgroup.org/news/group/generation-z-career-plans-and-expectations

SUPERPOWER 7

1   Alhola, P & Polo-Kantola, P 2007, 'Sleep Deprivation: Impact on cognitive performance', *Neuropsychiatric Disease and Treatment*, vol 3, no 5, pp 553-567, https://www.ncbi.nlm.nih.gov/pmc/articles/PMC2656292

2   Nutt, D, Wilson, S, & Paterson, L 2008, 'Sleep disorders as core symptoms of depression' *Dialogues in Clinical Neuroscience*, vol 10, no 3, pp 329-336, https://pubmed.ncbi.nlm.nih.gov/18979946

3   Matthews, G, 2020, Goals Research Summary, PDF, Dominican University of California, California,

4   Roosevelt, T 1910, *Citizenship In A Republic*, speech delivered at the Sorbonne, in Paris, France, 23 April 1910.

SUPERPOWER 9

1   Clement, J 2021, *Gamification Market Value Worldwide 2016-2021*, webpage, Statista, https://www.statista.com/statistics/608824/gamification-market-value-worldwide

2   McDonigal, J 2012, *Reality is Broken: Why games make us better and how they can change the world*, Random House, UK.

EPILOGUE

1   Merriam-Webster. (n.d.). Metamorphosis. In Merriam-Webster.com dictionary. Retrieved May 12, 2022, from https://www.merriam-webster.com/dictionary/metamorphosis

Notes

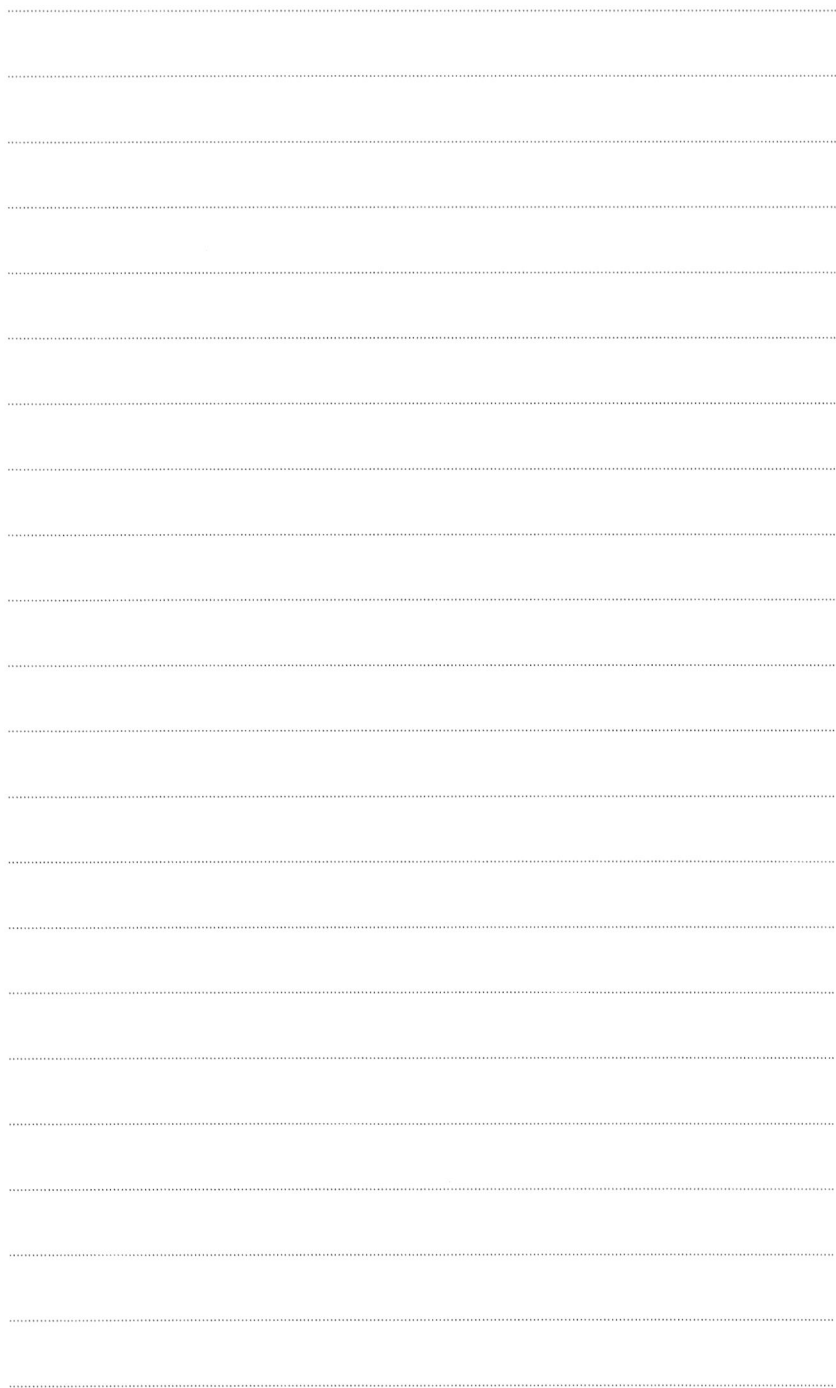

Are you ready to dive deep into your personal development?

If you're ready for real transformation but just need a little extra support and direction, then grab a copy of my workbook and start the real work with me as your guide.

The workbook is a personal journey of self-enquiry and awareness that will help you remove old mental blocks and behaviours and form new healthy beliefs and behaviours for positive outcomes.

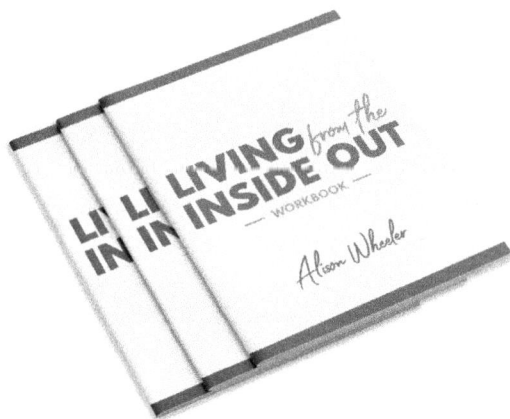

GRAB YOUR COPY AT
THEALISONWHEELER.COM/THE-BOOK

I look forward to working with you.

www.ingramcontent.com/pod-product-compliance
Lightning Source LLC
Chambersburg PA
CBHW062125020426
42335CB00013B/1103